NO-NONSENSE GUIDE TO

PSYCHIATRIC DRUGS

Including Mental Effects of Common Non-Psych Medications

A SmartMEDinfo book by

Moira Dolan, M.D.

No-Nonsense Guide to Psychiatric Drugs
Including Mental Effects of Common Non-Psych Medications
A SmartMEDinfo Book
By Moira Dolan, M.D.

For more about this author please visit http://www.smartmedinfo.com.

Ordering Information:

Quantity sales. Special discounts are available on quantity purchases by corporations, associations, and others. Orders by U.S. trade bookstores and wholesalers. For details, contact the publisher through http://www.smartmedinfo.com.

Disclaimer:

The information provided here is an interpretation of information that is made generally available to the physician. This is not intended to be a comprehensive nor exhaustive review of everything known in any quarter about the topics and it is not medical advice. It is provided as a supplement to patient/doctor discussions in order to facilitate informed consent. Patients are advised to consult with their trusted health care practitioner if they are considering changes in their medication regimen.

Editing services provided by The Pro Book Editor
Interior design services provided by Indie Author Publishing Services
Cover design by Alex Croft

ISBN: 978-0-9968860-0-0
Main category—Reference>Consumer Guides
Other category—Health & Fitness>Health Care Issues
Printed in the United States of America
First Edition

OTHER BOOKS

No-Nonsense Guide to Cholesterol Medications, Informed Consent and Statin Drugs

No-Nonsense Guide to Antibiotics, Dangers, Benefits & Proper Use

Dedicated to the memory of Thomas Szasz, M.D., the original plain-speaking author in the field of psychiatric informed consent.

TABLE OF CONTENTS

CHAPTER 1

Why Get Informed About Psychiatric Drugs?

In order to weigh the risks and benefits and make a rational decision about taking pscyhiatric drugs it is necessary to be aware of peritnent information.

What is a psychiatric drug?

How do psychiatric drugs act on the body and mind?

What is known and not known about how effective psychiatric treatments are?

What is known and not known about the safety and hazards of psychiatric drugs?

What are the alternatives to psychiatric drugs?

What are the potential or actual conflicts of interest between the entities recommending and selling psychiatric drugs?

The purpose of this book is to assist you in achieving enough information to support your *Informed Consent*. The legal defintion of Informed Consent is a situation "whereby a person can be said to have given consent based upon a full appreciation and understanding of the facts and implications of any actions, with the individual being in possession of all of his faculties (not mentally retarded or mentally deranged), and his judgment not being impaired at the time of consenting (by sleepiness, intoxication by alcohol or drugs, other health problems, etc.)."[1]

But it is almost never mental incompetence that inhibits rational medical decision-making. The failure to logically challenge the necessity for a prescription can be the result of social pressures such as fear of ridicule for questioning popular medical trends, or the time pressure of a usual seven-minute patient-doctor face to face visit. The usual patient is more likely to grill his auto mechanic on the need for a brake job than he is to question the workability and side effects of the powerfully mind altering drugs he is being prescribed. The opportunity for true informed consent is lacking for nearly any prescription doled out in a doctor's office, but it is most conspicuously absent when pscyhiatric drugs are prescribed. In that setting, any doubt expressed by the patient can be interpreted as disputing the authority of the physician—daring to defy the doctor. There is an implied threat of being labelled *non-compliant* for questioning doctor's orders or, worse, labeled as even more *mentally ill.*

Most of the time, the lack of Informed Consent is based on just plain ignorance, on the part of the patient and the physician. Physicians in a busy managed-care practice do not routinely go home and read their medical journals, and rarely ever do so with a critical eye. Most doctors do not challenge the latest drug news as supplied by pharmaceutical marketing divisions. And sadly, most patients do not know about their legal right to Informed Consent.

Physicians are ethically and legally obliged to facilitate Informed Consent. Medical ethics is a concept dating back at least to Hippocrates, a Greek physician born between 470 and 460 BC. His writings are the earliest Greek medical documents known and include the famous Hippocratic Oath: a set of instructions to newly trained physicians on their expected professional behavior. There are many translations of what is believed to be the original oath written by Hippocrates. Classical versions are an oath to the gods and include promises to honor your teacher, pass on your medical knowledge, apply nutritional remedies, refrain from using or suggesting deadly drugs, refuse to participate in abortion, leave surgery to the surgeons, vow to never engage in sexual relations with a patient, and to maintain confidentiality. Many medical schools have taken the liberty of modifying the oath by dropping the opening vow to the gods, omitting any reference to the prohibition against abortion, and qualifying the ban on sexual activity with patients. It is generally interpreted as simply keeping the patients' best interests at heart. [2]

The oath has been popularly summarized as "first do no harm," which is a phrase that does not actually appear in the classical version. The promise to refrain from using deadly drugs is the predecessor to modern Informed Consent, though there is no mention of discussing risks and benefits with the patient. Knowing all drugs have some potential for adverse effects, how does today's physician adhere to the oath to refrain from giving or suggesting deadly drugs? The practice of providing for Informed Consent is the closest we come to really following this ethical code.

Medical ethics codes through the 19th century strictly dealt with the physician's opinion of what he thought was best for the patient. Obtaining a patient's consent was not addressed directly until the aftermath of WWII. The Nuremberg Trials included testimony on atrocities committed by the Nazis in the name of medical science. Criminal proceedings were held for 23 physicians and administrators who carried out political objectives of the Nazi regime on the thin pretext of so-called medical treatments, including racial murder (eugenics), euthanasia (killing off the unwanted), and medical experimentation until the subject died. The court's proceedings heard 85 witnesses and evaluated some 1,500 records kept by the Nazi doctors. While the findings of criminality focused on the deeds committed in the course of "acts of duty" during wartime, the investigation encompassed civilian and pre-war conduct as well.

In response to the findings, the Nuremberg Directives for Human Experimentation were composed, usually referred to as the *Nuremberg Code.* The Code specifies that participants can consent to human experimentation only after full information is communicated and they have been given an opportunity to evaluate it. The Code states that consent should be entirely voluntary in that it should be free of coercion. The medical information should be given in a way that is easily understandable and prepared with the intention of truly enlightening the potential participant. It should clearly spell out "all inconveniences, hazards...and effects on his health or person" that may result from the treatment. [3]

The next advance in Informed Consent was the Declaration of Helsinki, a policy of the World Medical Association. It was first adopted in 1964 in Helsinki, Finland and revised many times since. The Declaration modernizes the concepts dealt with in the Nuremberg Code and expands on the basic principles. It addresses ethical standards that promote respect for all human beings and protect their health and rights during human experimentation. It calls for subjects to be consenting volunteers as informed participants. [4]

The phraseology in the Helsinki Declaration extends the concept of experimentation to include the usual practice of clinical medicine. It implies that there can be perhaps unintended, disregarded, covert or overt human experimentation well outside of the bounds of a research program; for example, *off-label* applications. This means giving a drug for something or to someone other than what or who the country's drug regulating agencies approved it for. In the US, the Food and Drug Administration (FDA) is the national drug regulating body. The Helsinki Declaration has been cited when drugs for off-label applications have been prescribed in the absence of Informed Consent—that is, the patient was not told by the doctor that the FDA did not approve the drug for his or her condition, gender, or age group. An example of off-label would be the psychiatric drug Effexor being prescribed for migraine headaches when it is only approved for depression. In that case, the doctor is supposed to tell the patient his prescription amounts to an experiment.

The Belmont Report is a uniquely American informed consent code. It expressly includes behavioral medical interventions, meaning psychiatric and psychological treatment of all kinds. It emphasizes that the patient is to be given adequate information on risks and benefits conveyed in a way so as to be fully understood by the patient, and any consent to treatment must be entirely voluntary. The implication in the Belmont Report is that a person is not really voluntarily consenting to treatment when he or she has not been given adequate information with which to make such a decision. [5]

The responsibility of Informed Consent means doctors are supposed to obtain a person's agreement to any course of treatment, and in order to do so, they must tell the patient anything that may substantially affect the patient's decision.

The information provided here is the same information that is made generally available to the physician, but which most physicains do not bother to pass on to their patients. This is not intended to be a comprehensive nor exhaustive review of everything known in any quarter about mentioned drugs. It is provided to empower the patient in intiating the informed consent conversation. I am obliged to state that it should be used as supplement to patient/doctor discussions, although this book actually contains more information than you are likely to ever get from your doctor.

CHAPTER 2

ORIGINS OF PSYCHIATRY

To understand terms related to psychiatry, it is worthwhile to look at the word root *psyche*, which comes from 17th century Latin origin when it meant "the human soul, the animating spirit" and Greek origin meaning "the invisible animating principle or entity which occupies and directs the physical body; the soul, mind, spirit, breath, life; understanding." It wasn't until the 20th century that psyche referred commonly only to "the mind." By the mid-20th century rise in biological psychiatry, the concept of "the mind" was largely replaced with "the brain," making it a medical field focusing on mental disorders in terms of biological cause and effect.

A psychiatric treatment is anything applied with the intention of affecting thinking, mood, emotion, or behavior. The mainstay of psychiatric treatment is the prescription drug although physical brain modalities, such as electroshock, are making a quiet comeback. [1]

Related terms:

- *psychotropic* – from psyche + *tropic*, originating from the Greek tropikos: "relating to a turn or change"; hence, that which turns the mind.

- *psychoactive* – a substance which affects the mind by virtue of being chemically active in the brain; psychoactive substances include any prescribed psychiatric medications, as well as medications given for another reason that may have psychotropic side effects. Psychoactive substances include mind-altering street drugs, newly synthesized chemicals, and even traditional plants and alcohol.

The concept of psyche is stretched even further in the medical field today known as biological psychiatry, which is an entire system explaining behaviors as responses to physical triggers, with the cornerstone being brain biochemistry. As described on the website of the Society of Biological Psychiatry, it uses a "medical model"—a term referring to conceiving of disorders relating to the physical body, in which non-psychiatric doctors are trained. The medical model addresses the patient's physical complaints by taking a medical history, conducting a thorough physical examination, obtaining ancillary tests if needed, and making a diagnosis based on all of this data, then offering a validated treatment. Biological psychiatry emulates the science of physical medicine in its medical terminology and appearances, and represents itself as a branch of physical medicine. This is made easier by the fact that there is a division of physical medicine called *neurology* (the study of the nervous tissue and brain). A conventional neurologist deals with physical brain diseases such as seizures and strokes. [2]

If the source of all mental and spiritual distress is assigned to the brain, it becomes easy to link it to neurology. Thus, by incremental steps, psychiatry morphs itself into a specialty dealing with physically-based disorders, and eventually thoroughly mimics a real medical paradigm.

Psychiatry does its theorizing, research, and publishing so thoroughly using this medical model that it is easy for practitioners to lose track of it being intended as only a model. They all-too-readily begin to believe the intangibles of humankind such as faith, love, and hate are physically based entities and that spiritual well-being (or distress) is determined by genes, brain structure, and molecular biochemical reactions. But the converse is also claimed: influences of culture, family, and physical environment are described as exerting their effects by way of shaping brain structure and biochemistry. In all of this, there is no allowance for individual personality, much less opinion or imagination.

An indirect suggestion that behavioral problems were of a physical nature came from observations of various plant toxicities and poisonings. Examples: [3]

- Lead used in making the wines consumed in ancient Rome has been attributed to the crazy behaviors of the ruling class culminating in the fall of their civilization.
- Chronic mercury exposure was known to cause insanity in miners and felters (memorably depicted in the character of the Mad Hatter in *Alice's Adventures in Wonderland*).
- Chewed leaves of the khat plant caused exhilaration, and 13th century Arab physicians might have used the plant as a remedy for depression.
- South American Indians saw that the bark of the Ayahuasca vine caused a hallucinogenic trip.
- The Asian poppy has been cultivated since recorded history for its sedative effects.

There was also abundant evidence of physical events resulting in mental afflictions:

- Stroke and head trauma could affect mood, emotion, and behavior.
- Sailors on long trips were at risk of becoming deficient in niacin (vitamin B3) that manifested as the four Ds: dermatitis, diarrhea, dementia, and death.
- Some people were never right in the head after illnesses with fever.
- It was observed since the late 15th century arrival of syphilis on European shores that some people went mad in the later stage of the disease.

Immediately before the modern era of biological psychiatry, the size and shape of the brain and skull were presented as a legitimate science of the mind. The study of head contour was called *phrenology* (from *phren* "mind" + *ology* "study of"). Phrenologists would palpate the head and thus "read" it, identifying bumps that informed them about the subject's personality and disposition. For example, a phrenology guide dated 1844 advised what head contours made a person prone to excessive sexual activity, argumentative, deceitful, or cowardly, or suitable only for a clerical profession. [4]

Legitimacy of assigning a physical basis to mental symptoms was boosted by the discovery in the mid-1800s of the cause of malaria (*mal* "bad" + *aria* "air"), a disease that frequently caused mental symptoms, particularly depression. Malaria was originally thought to be caused by bad air coming off the marshlands, but is actually caused by a parasite transmitted by mosquitos, which then lives on in human red blood cells.

The biological psychiatry movement was catalyzed by the 1906 discovery of the bacteria that causes syphilis. Syphilis is a sexually transmitted disease that starts with skin ulcers and progresses to a second stage of infection in lymph nodes and internal organs. In the late stage of syphilis, the brain and nerves are infected and it can cause confusion, depression, poor concentration, and, eventually, insanity. So here was proof in the modern era that infections affecting the brain caused insanity.

One psychiatrist thought perhaps it would be helpful to "superimpose one disease on another." Julius Wagner-Jauregg actually won a Nobel Prize in Medicine in 1927 for reporting that syphilitic insanity improved in 6 out of 9 people after he infected them with blood taken from a person in the throes of high fever from malaria. Fever therapy became popular even though far less than half of patients improved significantly; many of those only had temporary relief, and of course some died of malaria. Wagner-Jauregg was not a kind man: his hobby as a small child was to dissect animals, he was a Nazi party member, and he advocated for the sterilization of all persons labeled mentally ill and those with "criminal genes." In another effort to treat like with like, he subjected shell-shocked WWI veterans to electroshock, for which he was eventually put on trial for maltreatment of patients. [5]

Another boost for biological psychiatry came in 1958 when it was discovered on autopsy that certain areas of the brain of patients with Parkinson's disease had lost the cells that manufacture the biochemical dopamine. While the original descriptions of Parkinson's focused only on tremors and stiffness and did not include any mental symptoms, it was the first linkage of an inherent biochemical deficiency with a distinct brain disorder. Biological psychiatry had found its scientific foothold at last.

Psychiatry strives to identify which physical abnormalities result in what particular flavor of insanity. However, any actual discoveries of this sort make the underlying disease a truly medical one by definition, therefore taking it out of the realm of psychiatry. The most obvious example is Parkinson's disease. Syphilis and niacin deficiency are other examples. In all three, there are anatomic or biochemical abnormalities clearly identified, making them true medical illnesses.

Psychiatry fails spectacularly when it tries to pinpoint which brain structures, genes, and biochemicals result in specific unwanted behaviors. On the other hand, what psychiatry succeeds at is identifying psychoactive modalities that themselves most definitely affect brain structures, biochemicals, and behavior.

CHAPTER 3

PSYCHIATRIC NAMING

The leap from naming something to regarding that name as a diagnosis is a huge one, and this is where the "model" breaks down. In physical medicine there are definite objective signs that can be observed and measured, such that no matter who made the observation or measurement they would conclude the same diagnosis as anyone else making an observation. In contrast, psychiatric diagnoses are based on how the observer feels about the behavior he is facing. One person may call the behavior attention deficit disorder, while another may consider it is attention deficit hyperactivity disorder and another decide it is an expression of normal childhood. This is understandable since unlike medical illness, there is no objective test to prove whether the person in question has the named psychiatric condition or not. It has been said that mental illness is the only diagnosis requiring two people: one to exhibit the behavior, the other to call it abnormal. In contrast, if a diabetic were alone on a deserted island his blood sugar would still be abnormal even if no one were there to witness it.

Nomenclature is the devising or choosing of names for things.

The history of psychiatric nomenclature is a fascinating reflection of the struggles of psychiatry to establish itself as a legitimate medical science. Psychiatric labels are presented as being equivalent to medical diagnoses. Terms for unwanted behaviors would have to convey the notion of an "illness" in order for the practice of psychiatry to consistently emulate the medical model. Naming a behavior as an illness puts it exclusively in the camp of medicine because an illness naturally calls for a doctor and justifies the medical profession claiming authority over the subject.

The nomenclature experts in psychiatry meet on a recurring basis to re-fashion and add to their vocabulary. Their current naming book, the *Diagnostic and Statistical Manual (DSM)*, is a list of labels called "disorders." In other words, the *DSM* is a book of lists. The lists of disorders with no tests to validate them are a definite concession to the fact that characterizing moods, emotions, and behaviors as true illnesses or diseases cannot be substantiated in the way that medical conditions are documented.

The history of naming human behaviors would be entertaining if it did not imply severe consequences for so-labeled individuals and groups. The word *hysteria*, for instance, originates in ancient Greece as *hystera*, meaning "uterus" and was believed to be a disorder exclusive to women for at least 2,000 years. [1] At many times in history, a wandering womb or displaced uterus was figured to be the cause of almost all that could afflict a woman, but especially her mood changes and any other behaviors to which a male-dominated society might object. So-called hysteria has historically been treated by prescribing sex, prescribing abstinence, fumigating the vagina with foul herbs, and administration of herbal tonics of varying toxicities. In the year 2 AD, the anatomist Galen recommended that marriage could at times affect a complete cure. In the Middle Ages, the treatment for women labeled hysterical took a malicious turn: they were subjected to exorcism or tried by Inquisition panels, then burned as witches.

By the 17th century in Europe, the mood changes of women began to be attributed to brain and nerve problems that only secondarily affected the womb. An 18th century physician popularized the concept that hysteria arose when a woman deviated from normally expected womanly roles in the home and society. *Furor uterinus* (literally, rage of the womb) became the Latinized version of the same affliction in the Victorian era. By the mid-19th century, hysteria was considered an inherited, degenerative neurologic disease and was diagnosed in men as well as women. The concept of hysteria in men was popularized by Freud, who even diagnosed it in himself. Military hospitals of World War I catalogued hysteria as a prevalent diagnosis among soldiers, but the same symptoms were given alternate labels *anxiety* and *conversion disorder* in World War II hospitals.

There was a further decline in the use of the word *hysteria* in the second half the 20th century, and by 1980 it was dropped altogether by the *Diagnostic and Statistical Manual (DSM).* The *DSM* now catalogues symptoms once called *hysterical* as part of *dissociative disorder.* [2]

The many names assigned to "the blues" parallels the history of difficulties in attaching a physical cause to mental distress.

The ancients considered overall health to result from an optimal balance of four liquids circulating in the body (called "humours" [3]): blood, phlegm, black bile, and yellow bile. Bile is digestive fluid made by the liver and concentrated in the gall bladder, from where it passes into the gut to aid fat absorption. Excess or deficiency, infection or decay of any one of the four humours was thought to result in disease states that could have physical and mental manifestations.

Ancient Greeks described *melancholia* as a perpetual gloominess, a feeling of sadness and despair, feeling grief or loss. The word derives from *melas* "black" + *khole* "bile"; literally excess of black bile. [4] Animal dissections were done to discover the source of the bad mood, although it is unclear how they could tell goats or pigs were depressed. In later centuries, dissections of human bodies likewise could not demonstrate the defective humour or pinpoint the physical cause of melancholia. In contrast, philosophers throughout the ages described melancholia in all of its forms, not as disease, but simply as part of the normal human experience of being alive.

In 1621, Robert Burton wrote *The Anatomy of Melancholy* as a medical textbook. It was subtitled: *What it is: With all the Kinds, Causes, Symptomes, Prognostickes, and Several Cures of it. In Three Maine Partitions with Their Several Sections, Members, and Subsections. Philosophically, Medicinally, Historically, Opened and Cut Up*. He provided in-depth explanations of melancholy, not only based on the popular psychological and physiologic notions of the time, but also ranging from astronomy and astrology to theology and demonology. It is much more entertaining than reading the *DSM*, but similarly brimming with invented nomenclature. [5]

By the eighteenth century, the description of melancholia became more generalized. *Hypochondria* was a related term, from *hypo* "under" + *khondros* "cartilage," indicating the anatomic location of the source of the foul vapors causing the bad mood. Hypochondria came to mean having symptoms for which there was no medical explanation. Sometimes, sad mood was simply called *vapors*. Eventually, sufferers were described as *splenic*; it is not clear if black bile was thought to emanate from the spleen (a fist-sized organ tucked under the left-sided ribs), or if the whole black bile concept was gradually replaced with blaming depression on defective blood-filtering by the spleen. [6]

In the 19th century, the physical sciences were making great strides:

- in 1801 the word biology was introduced, from French *biologie;* from *bio* "life" + *logy* "study of";
- the stethoscope was invented;
- electricity was measured for the first time;
- Charles Darwin proposed his theory of *evolution,* which was a new use of the word;
- it was proven that germs caused disease and Louis Pasteur invented the process of heating milk to kill bacteria (*pasteurization).*
- the agent responsible for a disease of tobacco plants was named a *virus.*

The century provided an explosion of scientific terminology, including the modern system for naming chemical compounds, the taxonomy of classifying plants, a revised and expanded nomenclature for anatomy, and a vocabulary for the study of inheritance.

The newly invented specialty of psychiatry was not going to be left out of the naming frenzy, and most of the new psychiatric names referred to a supposed physical cause of the disorder. In that era, what we know as depression was called *neurasthenia,* a weakness of nerves (from *neuro* "nerve" + *a* "without" + *sthenos* "strength"). *Dysthymia* was an alternate word referring to a supposedly causative poorly functioning thyroid gland or thymus gland, which are two organs that modulate metabolism.

Emil Kraeplin and Sigmund Freud were both born in 1856 and became psychiatrists. While Freud's name is still cited in popular culture, few outside of psychiatric circles know of Kraeplin, who turned out to have far more influence on modern psychiatry than Freud. Kraeplin's life work was concentrated on forwarding psychiatry as a valid physical medical science. He advanced the notion that naming the condition was equal to diagnosis of disease. To this end, he popularized the theory of physical brain degeneration being the cause of mental illness.

The remarkable lack of physical evidence for this theory did not seem to be a concern to Kraeplin and his followers. In lieu of actual evidence, he created psychiatric names for various behaviors in terms that were acceptable to physicians. Furthermore, the terms sounded very scientific to the lay public. Kraeplin's first edition of *Compendium der Psychiatrie* was published in 1883 and introduced the term *manic-depressive insanity.* Specifically, he considered mania and depression to be alternate expressions of one single affliction. He described mental problems as a spectrum from mildly abnormal to severely disturbed, with no clear distinctions along the way. Kraeplin introduced the term *dementia praecox,* literally "brain degeneration starting at an early age." The cases he described would later be called *schizophrenia.* [7]

Kraeplin was also a promoter of *eugenics,* which is controlled breeding and selective killing in order to create a supposedly superior race. He was a fan of social Darwinism—a political theory that argues superior inheritance results in the success of the most fit in human society. Kraeplin advanced the notion that Jews, among other non-Aryan races, carried biological factors that made them prone to degenerative brain disorders resulting in mental illness. These concepts provided key pseudo-scientific support to the foundations of the Nazi racial hygiene programs. In 1917, Kraeplin established the German Research Institute for Psychiatry that was later affiliated with the Kaiser Wilhelm Society for the Advancement of Science; it served as the breeding ground for the psychiatric programs carried out by Hitler's regime. [8]

Kraeplin ceaselessly expanded his lists to include a classification system grouping patterns of symptoms and behaviors; the more he observed, the more numerous were the human conditions that appeared to be abnormal to him, so he had to keep coming up with names. Kraeplin was described by historians as having a quirk for novelty, and he was certainly prolific in his invention of new words and phrases. [9]

Mental retardation, criminality, epilepsy, homelessness, and prostitution were all considered by Kraeplin to be psychiatric disorders originating in brain disease. By the time of his tenth edition (published after his death), his description of psychiatric maladies consisted of four volumes and was ten times larger than the first edition. Not everyone embraced Kraeplin's naming scheme; however, it did open the door for anyone to jump in and likewise invent names. Meanwhile, in America, the classification of mental afflictions was limited to a few terms: dementia, *dipsomania* (alcoholism) epilepsy, mania, melancholia, *monomania* (obsessive enthusiasm about a single topic), and *paresis* (another term for the insanity caused by syphilitic brain infection).

The American Medico-Psychological Association established their spin on the terminology in 1918. Their stated purpose was to assist the US Census Bureau in collecting statistics on citizens locked up in insane institutions. In the first version of the *Statistical Manual for the Use of Institutions for the Insane*, nearly every condition is called a *psychosis.* At that time, the word meant any mental derangement, which is a profound perversion of the root word from the Greek *psykhosis* that meant "a giving of life; animation; principle of life." Their 22 groupings included Kraeplin's dementia praecox and his manic-depressive psychosis, but also listed something called "constitutional psychopathic inferiority," which implies there was something inherent in the person's body that made him nuts. It also described a purely depressed state as "involutional melancholia." These fanciful terms were alongside of mental conditions well-established as due to actual physical causes like the deficiency of vitamin B3 (*pellagra)*, traumatic head injury, brain tumor or stroke, drugs and toxins, and syphilis of the brain. This manual also established a convenient tradition that would be expanded greatly and remains in major use today: they had a listing called "Unknown Psychosis" and various sub-categories simply called "Other." [10]

The manual went through ten editions during which time the Medico-Psychological Association recreated itself as the American Psychiatric Association (APA), largely to differentiate from psychologists (who were not medical doctors). The terminology of these organizations is of interest. Both psychology and psychiatry are based on the root word *psych* "the human soul; animating spirit"; psychology adds – *ology* "the study of," while psychiatry adds – *iatry*, from *iatros* "treatment" or "healing." Literally then, psychology would be the study of the soul, while psychiatry would be the treatment of the soul. This differentiation underscored the thrust of modern psychiatry away from talk therapy and into a focus on brain-altering modalities. Both professions insist they are dealing primarily with the brain and biochemicals.

A 1946 US War Department Technical Bulletin called *Medical 203*, developed by Brigadier General and psychiatrist William Menninger, represents the next level of complexity in psychiatric naming. *Medical 203* grouped behaviors into descriptions of a multitude of "reactions." For example, the category of Immaturity Reactions applied to "physically adult individuals who are unable to maintain their emotional equilibrium and independence under minor or major stress." *Medical 203* had a distinct section for Organic Psychosis, which were "psychoses with demonstrable etiology or associated structural changes." This category included syphilitic psychosis, vitamin deficiencies, post-stroke dementia, and remains in the latest version of the *DSM* today, which underscores the fact that the majority of the "disorders" still do not have a demonstrable etiology or associated structural change. [11] Any condition reliably demonstrated to be caused by physical factors is automatically the concern of usual medicine, and it does not belong in the scope of psychiatry.

The first edition of the American Psychiatric Association's *Diagnostic and Statistical Manual (DSM)* in 1952 adopted much from *Medical 203* while carrying forward a lot of Kraeplin's terminology as well. [12] Its construction was fascinatingly arbitrary: a writing committee of the APA sent a draft to just 10% of its members, of which less than half replied. 93% of the respondents gave their approval, and after more work-overs by the committee, the first edition of the *DSM* was published. It listed 106 mental disorders. *DSM-I* was criticized for failing to identify a distinct boundary between normal human emotions and abnormal mental states. This slight little problem was never fixed, and the exact same criticism is leveled at the newest version of the *DSM* today. In the 1968 version called *DSM-II* "involutional melancholia" was still there, but somehow manic-depressive reactions became manic-depressive illness, with no medical evidence submitted to substantiate the switch. [13]

Major revisions appeared in *DSM-III* (1980) [14] and *DSM-III-R* (1987) [15]; the latter was 567 pages and included 292 diagnoses. It expanded on the idea of the undefined category "Other" by adding listings for "Not Otherwise Specified" (NOS) at the end of most of its categories. That way, the NOS designation could be applied whenever a person did not fit into any of the 292 descriptions. This most revealing statement was in the preface of *DSM-III-R*:

"...there is no assumption that each mental disorder is a discrete entity with sharp boundaries between it and other mental disorders or between it and no mental disorder." [15]

That quote deserves re-reading if it did not sink in for you.

The authorities on mental health are admitting they cannot differentiate one condition from another or from no mental disorder. This would be hilarious if the *DSM* were not the basis for involuntary commitment, child custody decisions, and avoiding responsibility for violent crimes and immoral acts. In her book *Whores of the Court*, psychologist Margaret Hagen explains how the *DSM* is nothing more than "science by decree." We are asked to believe if it is described and written as a diagnosis, then it is to be accepted as if it were science without any intervening evidence validating the pronouncement. [16]

By the time of *DSM-IV* in 1994, the book was 866 pages long and listed nearly 300 disorders, even though it deleted some old ones. Some notable additions included sexual aversion disorder and sexual addiction, although no mention is made of penis envy—the term used by Freud. One of the most controversial additions was childhood bipolar disorder. In Europe, it is not legitimate to diagnose a child as bipolar, since they consider daily ups and downs to be part of normal childhood. [17]

In 2000, the text revision of the fourth edition of the *DSM (DSM-IV-TR)* offered another disclaimer: "...no definition adequately specifies precise boundaries for the concept of 'mental disorder'."[18]

DSM-V (2013) added 15 new disorders, including Internet gaming disorder, hoarding disorder, and cannabis withdrawal, but dropped sexual aversion disorder and categorized first time drug users with drug addicts. Disruptive mood dysregulation disorder finally gives a medical-sounding name to temper tantrums. Delirium, schizophrenia, and panic disorder are listed as brain diseases with no evidence to support this classification. "Unspecified" replaces "Not Otherwise Specified" as a catchall, in case a person's objectionable behavior defies description.

The criteria for making a mental diagnosis in *DSM-V* so obviously attempts to medicalize everyday life experience that it has become a subject of intense criticism. For example, in earlier versions, the diagnosis of major depressive disorder used to exclude anyone who was grieving the recent loss of a loved one. That exclusion has since been removed and anyone who is still feeling grief more than two weeks after attending a funeral is now certifiably mentally ill. [19] Paul McHugh, a professor and former psychiatrist-in-chief at Johns Hopkins Hospital, says *DSM-V* is more of a checklist than a diagnostic guide and likens it to a naturalist's field guide to the birds. [20]

In a discussion of the uselessness of *DSM-V* in his online blog, the Director of the National Institute for Mental Health, Dr. Thomas Insel says, "We need to begin collecting the genetic, imaging, physiologic, and cognitive data to see how all the data—not just the symptoms—cluster and how these clusters relate to treatment response." [21]

Should we be comforted that the national director of a government agency which receives over $1.4 billion tax dollars annually would suggest that perhaps *beginning* to collect some data would be a good thing? Actual scientific backup is certainly an excellent concept for the basis of an entire profession and its *Diagnostic and Statistical Manual.* After all, this book provides justification for billing insurers billions of dollars per year, supports a multibillion-dollar pharmaceutical industry, and is the authorized reference manual in courts of law.

Who Actually Benefits From DSM-V?

Critics point to an unhealthy influence from the pharmaceutical industry on the revision process. Dr. Allen Frances, retired Duke University professor who headed the psychiatry group's task force and worked on the previous version, says *DSM-V* "would turn everyday anxiety, eccentricity, forgetting and bad eating habits into mental disorders." [22] The value of making an official diagnosis is that it comes with a billing code, which is a multi-digit number used to assure payment. The codes warrant not only billing for an office visit, but immediate and ongoing treatment, especially with drugs. All medical professionals—from allergists and family doctors to psychiatrists and urologists—are supposed to use the diagnostic codes in this manual to bill for services and prescriptions so they can be paid by insurance. This is why the *DSM* is commonly referred to as "the billing bible."

Persons not inclined to label themselves "mentally ill" may seek help from social workers, counselors or psychologists, not realizing that all mental health interactions now get recorded with a mental diagnosis code in order to get paid by insurance. These non-medical professionals are entering a *DSM* code for a mental diagnosis for every single visit, which becomes part of one's permanent medical record.

DSM-V was 14 years in the making, and an investigation in 2009 revealed most panel members had financial ties to pharmaceutical companies. [23] When there was an outcry about this, the panelists all vowed to sever ties from pharmaceutical companies, but they only did so for 12 months before the publication of the book. That 12 month period occurred after the writing of the material was completed and the content was already influenced by those ties. This temporary whitewash only reflects an extremely insincere concept of personal ethics in these psychiatrists. It also presumes the general public is so stupid as to be duped by their shady maneuvering. Find out more in the final chapter on conflict of interest.

Today's psychiatric drugs are named according to how they are marketed. If a drug is marketed for treatment of depression it is called an *antidepressant.* The same drug with a different brand name targets people who are quitting smoking, in which case it is called a *withdrawal agent.* Epilepsy drugs have been re-branded as *mood stabilizers.* Some drugs are named as an advertising gimmick with no basis in science, such as SSRI, which stands for Selective Serotonin Reuptake Inhibitors; the name gives the false idea that they selectively affect a brain biochemical called serotonin. Drugs given to violent people are called *antipsychotics*, although the same drugs used to be called *major tranquilizers*; in the institutional setting, they are simply referred to as *chemical straightjackets.*

Some psychiatric treatments are too gruesome to be called by their real names. For example, shock treatment was renamed *electroconvulsive therapy* (ECT). In another example, there was a specific kind of torture with the pleasant name of *aversion therapy*, in which allegedly deviant youths were given drugs to make them vomit while they were shown pornography and given electric shocks. [5]

The key to the prevalent acceptance of psychiatric naming is the degree of agreement regarding particular behaviors falling somewhere in the spectrum from just undesirable, all the way to absolutely unacceptable. In recent years, there is increasing agreement that more and more behaviors are entirely unacceptable, and corresponding willingness to embrace the solutions offered by psychiatry. Once upon a time, unacceptable behaviors included believing in one God. In another era, when all extended family members were contributing to the physical work of the farm, laziness was an unacceptable behavior. Independent behavior has often earned a psychiatric diagnosis, such as when the astronomer Galileo was labeled mentally ill because of reporting the earth revolved around the sun when "everybody knew" it was the other way around. The pattern here is that the larger society determines what is acceptable.

CHAPTER 4

A Brief History of Psychiatric Treatment

A psychiatric treatment is anything applied with the intention of affecting the mind (thinking), mood, emotion, or behavior. Today we almost never hear of old time talk therapy; the psychiatrist routinely neglects to explore negative influences in the home or to discuss effective coping mechanisms, changes of habit, or positive self-help modalities. Indeed, the modern psychiatrist is not even trained in these things.

Instead, the psychiatrist nearly exclusively pursues manipulation of the brain and brain chemicals. Their mainstay is the prescription drug, although direct physical brain treatments such as electroshock are making a quiet comeback.

As all modern day psychiatric treatment is physically based, it can derange brain function in many ways:

- impair memory;
- hamper the ability to learn;
- promote irrational decision-making;
- give weird concepts of self-identity;
- distort less well-defined qualities of a person's confidence, trust, and faith.

For a perspective on today's psychiatric practices it is useful to know that modern day treatments are only the latest in a long and gruesome tradition of man's attempts to suppress unwanted behaviors in his fellow man. The routine in psychiatric treatment has been the causation of harm in the name of help, intentional or not. For example, there is archeological evidence of 7,000 year old Neolithic societies using *trephining*, which is the practice of making an opening in the skull, often by drilling one or more holes. Anthropologists presume these represent treatments for mental problems because the human remains show evidence of otherwise totally healthy persons. [1] Written history of biological psychiatry extends to the ancient Greeks who administered the poison plant black hellebores to induce a purge (vomiting and diarrhea) in persons whose behaviors were rejected by society. [2]

Not all ancient remedies were so aggressive. Ancient healers following a more philosophical tradition recommended exercise for melancholia; a treatment that has been shown to be as effective as modern day antidepressant drugs when tested head to head. The ancients also advised warm baths, music, a regular sleep schedule, nutritious food, walks in nature, and taking up hobbies. Other treatments for mental distress included rituals performed with charms of astrological significance, and nearly every culture had its version of exorcism to free the victim of an elusive causative agent, spiritual or otherwise.

Those conservative approaches were frequently overshadowed by methods of addressing the body to drive out mental distress. Hundreds of concoctions have been offered up as cures for insanity, many causing vomiting and diarrhea in order to purge the victim of the bad humours. These included plants, oils, magnesium, and mercury. Bloodletting was episodically popular. Powdered rock crystals were tried. The dried carcass of the Spanish fly was applied to skin, raising blisters that were considered to be a sure sign of its effectiveness. It also happened to be an aphrodisiac, causing sexual arousal.

The basic paradigm is not very different from today's treatments. Instead of evil spirits or bad humours, prescription medications are supposed to be chasing down brain biochemical abnormalities that are causing bad thoughts. As you will learn in detail in the chapter on Prozac-like drugs, for example, it is only the advertising spin that has popularized serotonin deficiency as the "bad humour" of the day. And while we don't drill holes in the skull any more, we still apply electric shocks to an imagined but never measured brain wave problem in depressed people.

At one time, distilled snake venom was advertised to cure madness. It was originally concocted around 100 BC at the request of Methridates VI, the King of Pontus, in a region on the south coast of the Black Sea (modern day Turkey). The king feared his enemies would poison him as they had his father. At his direction, the king's shamans made preparations of diluted snake venom mixed with toxic herbs. The story is that Methridates became immune to poisons by taking small, diluted doses on a regular basis. The concoctions were later expanded to be preventative and serve as treatment for the bite of any wild animal. It came to be known as *theriac,* from the Greek word for "vicious animal." Later versions of theriac were mixed with opium or honey. Eventually it was doctored up as a patented formula containing additional herbs, minerals, and animal flesh and blood, and sold as a cure-all, especially for mental problems

Benjamin Rush is commonly referred to as the father of American psychiatry for forwarding the idea that mental distress was rooted in physical causes and offering "modern" medical treatments. The Pennsylvania-born Rush attended medical school in Scotland and wrote the first edition of his famous textbook in 1785 at the age of 39. In *Medical Inquiries and Observations Upon the Diseases of the Mind*, Rush rejected historical notions that madness was caused by bad bile or disorders of the digestion or internal organs. He also rejected that insanity was a nerve problem or a brain disease, because, he wrote, nerves and the brain were found to be normal on autopsies of dead mental patients. He stated, "I infer that madness is seated in the blood vessels," but offered no proof. Instead, he mentioned the tendency of the insane to have red eyes, a whitish tongue, and a "tense pulse." He even boasted that he was able to get the president to pardon a criminal by measuring his pulse to prove the convicted man was insane. Although Dr. Rush vaguely cited brain autopsies as supporting his theory, he went on to write that the brains of the insane show "absence of every sign of disease."

Rush's word for melancholia was *tristimania* (from Latin *tristis* meaning "sad, mournful, sorrowful, gloomy") and he created the term *menomania* for people who walked around with cheerful delusions. For both of these conditions, Rush recommended bloodletting and purges with herbs to cause diarrhea and vomiting, and/or mercury to cause excess salivation. His more aggressive remedies included warm baths followed by cold dunking and various means for causing pain, particularly by the burning of mustard preparations on abraded skin. The primary drug advised was *laudanum* (opium), which he called "a noble medicine."

Mania was the term Rush used to describe episodic periods of unusual preoccupation; he invented the word *manicula* to describe a low level, chronic form of mania, while *manglia* was used to describe such overwhelming mania that it reduced the person to being incapable of self-care.

Dr. Rush was no nice guy. "Terror," said Rush, "acts powerfully on the body through the medium of the mind, and should be employed in the cure of madness." He recommended confinement in an insane asylum and the application of "mild and terrifying modes of punishment." This consisted of restraint by straightjacket, tying to a chair that had a hole in the seat for bowel movements, shaving the head and affixing an ice-filled clay helmet, and pouring ice water down the straightjacket sleeves so it could run onto the body. More commonly, he said, the inmate thus tied in the so-called "tranquilizing chair" should be immersed in cold water for several hours. Today the straightjacket effect is achieved through chemical means with the so-called *neuroleptic* (brain seizing) drugs, as described in chapter 9.

Rush advised bloodletting in volumes of up to 40 ounces or until fainting, whichever occurred first. Forty ounces is a quarter of all the blood a person has, and today that much blood loss is recognized as Class II Hemorrhage, at which point the patient begins to go into shock. This was a precursor to 20th century insulin coma and electroshock therapy. Bloodletting was a common treatment for various physical ailments, but Rush advised greater quantities should be drained for mental afflictions than for any organic disease (actual physical illness). He bragged about patients from which he drained 200 ounces over less than three months and 740 ounces over ten months. At one point, Rush was accused of malpractice for his bloodletting enthusiasm, but he successfully countersued his accuser.

"Fear, accompanied with pain, and a sense of shame, has sometimes cured this disease," wrote Rush. In addition to the good-for-everything purges, mercury, and near starvation ("low diet"), other treatments included locking up inmates in a solitary dark cell and not allowing any light while forcing them to sit erect, tied to a chair, day and night. Exposure to sudden or constant loud sounds and various measures to induce great pain were also endorsed. For extreme cases, Rush described at length the benefits of a warm bath followed by being dunked in cold. He described one patient who recovered his senses from this regimen, but alas he died in his cell later from "pulmonary consumption" (pneumonia). Another treatment was to burn the back of the head and neck, creating open ulcers, then keep them open for years in order to drain the brain. One of Dr. Rush's notable special treatments was a gyrator to which the patient was strapped and spun and lurched about. Rush said he would resort to "a stroke or two of the whip or of the hand" only in case there was an "unprovoked" attack upon the physician. It is hard to imagine what would qualify as unprovoked in these situations.

Rush rejected common vulgar terms for some mental afflictions. He said people who were "flighty," "hair-brained," or "cracked in the head" should be called by the more medical sounding term *dissociative* to describe a loss of judgment. His terms for mental disorders were:

> dissociation,
>
> derangement of the will (addiction, drunkenness),
>
> derangements of faith (people who believe everything they hear),
>
> derangement of memory,
>
> diseases of *fatuity* (commonly referred to as idiocy), and
>
> derangement of passion of any kind (love, grief, excitement, fear).

They were all treated with purges, restricted calorie diet, bloodletting, and blistering. As a last resort, opium was a cure-all. Any mental upset could be treated by these means, according to Rush. Even dreaming, which Rush said "is a transient paroxysm of madness," and excessive laughter, which he said can "result in death" were categorized as mental illness. However, cures were rare. Mental patients lived in the Philadelphia Hospital for years.

Rush was a founding American, a signer of the Declaration of Independence, and a major influence in the developing American culture, but every one of his treatments were later abandoned. [3]

Fifty years after Dr. Rush, there was an effort to reverse the inhumanities used toward institutionalized persons. In one pamphlet issued for use by superintendents of insane asylums, the author John Galt urged adoption of more humane therapies in America modeled after a reformed asylum in England. In 1853, Galt wrote: "nine-tenths of the erroneous treatment of insanity has arisen from confounding insanity with phrenitis or inflammation of the brain, a disease requiring remedies usually contraindicated in the treatment of the insane..." In other words, actual physical inflammation of the brain such as from physical illnesses like meningitis or syphilis required the appropriate medical treatment, and afflicted persons should not be treated like mad men.

Galt represented the minority of health care professionals who did not think inmates were inherently defective. He suggested the institution should stock a reading library and provide calm, comfortable spaces for residents. He recommended supervised walks in the woods and neighborhood and plenty of encouragement for inmates to play cards and board games. Nevertheless, he endorsed opiates as the mainstay of treatment for "lulling excitement," especially "in continuous and considerable doses" and strongly objected to government regulation of opiate use and availability. [4]

Modest reforms were only embraced to a limited degree in some facilities. Twenty-five years later, a superintendent of Bethlehem Hospital documented his failures to cure mental patients with the use of chloral hydrate (knock-out fumes), with morphine for sedation, or with extract of the poisonous hemlock tree or various other drugs to cause purging. He concluded: "I would say that insanity requires no special treatment medicinally.... The moral treatment must for long, if not for ever, be the chief thing aimed at." The moral treatment he referred to is what we would call social and environmental: a safe, calm, and clean environment where recreation, hobbies, music, and exercise are encouraged. [5]

Despite efforts to introduce compassionate care, psychiatric treatment largely continued in the pattern of inducing shock by various means, combined with physical and chemical restraint.

Deep sleep therapy was introduced in the 1920s. It was achieved by injecting a combination of two *barbiturates* (strong sedatives) in order to put the body into a profoundly reduced metabolism resembling a death-like state. Patients were kept asleep for days at a time and it was popularized for weight loss—the Sleeping Beauty treatment was used by Elvis. The practice was later combined with electroshock and used for premenstrual symptoms, depression, and many other diagnoses. Deep drugging to induce near coma is still in sporadic use today despite exposes of criminal coercion, lack of informed consent, and patient deaths. [6]

Ladislas Joseph von Meduna was a Hungarian born psychiatrist who pointed out that very few people who were said to be schizophrenic also had a diagnosis of epilepsy. Through some bizarre twist of logic, he reasoned that causing seizures might cure the mental affliction. In the 1930s, Meduna experimented with various poisons (including strychnine) to cause seizures, and then found the stimulant drug metrazol best suited his aims; it caused an explosive seizure about a minute after injection. Meduna's initial reports of cures were not substantiated, but that did not dampen the widespread use of the procedure. [7]

Around the same time, insulin shock therapy came into vogue. It involved injecting insulin into non–diabetics to lower their blood sugar to such a level that the glucose-starved brain went into a coma. A usual course of treatment was 50 to 60 doses given in a closely timed series. Insulin coma was embraced by leading medical institutions of the day, but later thoroughly discredited. It is well established today that when diabetics who require insulin occasionally experience accidental overdoses of insulin, they are risking brain damage with each episode of severe *hypoglycemia* (low blood sugar). [8]

In the 1930s, the Portuguese psychiatrist and neurologist Antonio Moniz attended a medical lecture describing experiments involving brain surgery on two chimpanzees. Apparently they were more docile after the front lobes of their brains were removed. Moniz supposed that insane ideas travelled on defective nerves in the brain and sought to cut the connections to those nerves. He promoted this procedure even though he never identified any actual diseased brain or specific nerve abnormalities.

On his first patients, in 1935, Moniz drilled holes through the skull and injected alcohol to directly kill brain tissue. He soon refined the procedure by passing a thin wire-like knife to indiscriminately hash up random brain tissue. He called the practice *psychosurgery* (from *psyche* "soul" + *surgery* from *kheir* "hand" + *ergon* "work": *cutting of the soul*). The procedure soon came to be known as the *lobotomy.* In 1949, Moniz was recognized with a Nobel Prize for inventing psychosurgery.

Lobotomy was popularized in America by Walter Freeman and James Watts. The procedure was later modified to make it easier and faster: an icepick-like device was shoved under the brow and rammed into brain tissue where it was swiped back and forth to destroy the frontal lobe. In the 1950s, Freeman travelled around the country in his "lobotomobile" and offered the treatment as a cure for any mental distress. Meanwhile, Watts lobotomized the embarrassments of the rich and famous, including the 23-year old daughter of Joseph Kennedy. Death rates were high and, as best as can be discerned, agitated patients were simply turned into more agreeable, docile vegetables by the treatment. Rosemary Kennedy, like so many others who did not die on the table or within days of lobotomy, lived out her life as an insensible inmate of an institution. [9]

Concurrent to the lobotomy movement, Italian psychiatrist Ugo Cerletti (who had studied under Kraeplin) and his assistant Lucio Bini were busy with electroshock. They experimented by electro-shocking dogs, half of which died. They electroshocked their first human patient in 1938, and presented their supposed astonishingly successful results to the world. A careful review of Cerletti's papers revealed his accounts were pure fiction; Cerletti's reports of cures have been called no more than "an electroshock novel." [10]

Shock was first used in the US in 1940. Although the inventors and early users of the treatment called it "electroshock" or "electroconvulsive shock," it gradually came to be known by a kinder, gentler name of *electroconvulsive therapy*, or ECT. Jolts of electricity are coursed through the brain with the goal of intentionally creating a seizure. The orderly pattern of natural electrical activity of the brain is short-circuited by the shock, resulting in wildly chaotic brain activity that can be traced on a graph paper as rapid jagged lines.

In a person who is not anesthetized and paralyzed, the brain seizure would be accompanied by uncontrollable spasms of muscles, clenching of the jaw resulting in broken teeth and a bitten tongue, and violent arching of the back with such force as to cause spinal fractures. Electroshock is administered today while the patient is under anesthesia with paralyzed muscles to suppress the muscle jerking, which is the most recognizable part of a seizure. Modern ECT looks more benign, but in fact the electrical dosages are higher and the duration of the shocks are longer. [11] There is no consensus on what the mechanisms of action of ECT are, but especially with modern day drugs camouflaging the bodily effect, it is more acceptable to the public than lobotomy. A modern modification of electroshock is *deep brain stimulation*, in which wires are permanently implanted in the brain to deliver tiny electroshocks day and night.

Except for electroshock, all of the older physical therapies for mental conditions fell away rapidly upon introduction of the first chemical straightjackets. These were major tranquilizers introduced in the 1950s in the class known as *neuroleptic* drugs (from *neuro* "nerve or brain" + *leptic* "seize": "brain-seizing drugs"). Neuroleptics emerged out of research on veterinary anti-worming medications found to paralyze the nervous system of parasitic bugs. Modifications of the worming medications did not work on the malaria parasite as hoped, but researchers noticed the drugs made experimental animals sleepy and cooperative. [12]

When neuroleptics were introduced as psychiatric drugs for humans they were hailed as “agents of chemical lobotomy” because drugged patients were pleasantly blank and docile and gave their caretakers no trouble. These first generation drugs were rapidly popularized for all kinds of mental distress and went into broad use in society, not just in institutionalized persons. Neuroleptics were soon documented to cause severe adverse mental and physical effects.

Before neuroleptics, there were only two main classes of psychiatric drugs: sedatives such as barbiturates, opium, and morphine; and stimulants such as amphetamines. The advent of the neuroleptics and a population ready to consume them combined to launch the modern era of experimentation into all manner of drugs to affect brain biochemistry.

CHAPTER 5

Psychiatric Drugs and Your Brain

Contrary to popular myth, humans use much more than a small part of their brains. Although it is true that when certain regions of the brain are severely damaged specific neurologic deficits might result, the fact is that distinct human activities involve connections amongst multiple regions of the brain and not just one or two isolated areas. It was once taught that brain growth is complete by age 2, but it is now known that the brain adds new cells throughout life, including during old age. The brain is capable of self-repair to a great degree. It is extremely efficient, using the equivalent of only about 20 watts of energy to operate. No one knows how the brain manages to do this. It is estimated that if a computer could be built to match the most rudimentary functions of a human brain, it would consume a gigawatt of power—enough electricity to run a medium-sized city.

The brain has very strong protective mechanisms. It is encased in a thick bony box of a skull and can only be accessed through a blood-brain barrier, which under normal conditions allows for the controlled passage of only those substances necessary for life. For its size, the brain has impressive capacity to withstand impacts and electrical shocks. [1]

Any substance that affects the brain must have two key properties:

(1) It has to be similar enough to innate biochemicals such that the substance does not get recognized as a poison and therefore immediately rejected by the body (by vomiting or diarrhea).

(2) It has to penetrate the blood-brain barrier.

For a substance to be used as a medication, it has to have the additional qualities of first, not killing the patient outright, and second, causing a somewhat predictable reaction. As we will see, *indirectly* causing death is considered an acceptable feature of a medication. Examples of delayed toxicity considered acceptable are drug-induced mood changes leading to suicide or drug-induced diabetes leading to premature death.

The brain's normal biochemicals, named *neurotransmitters*, interact with brain cells to turn on, speed up, slow down, or turn off various cellular reactions. The amount and activity of neurotransmitters can be ramped up or toned down by many factors including temperature, exercise, sleep, sunlight, thoughts, emotions, hormones, stress, injury, pain, pleasure, hunger, infection, and psychoactive drugs.

Neurotransmitters all have *receptors* on brain cells. This refers to a configuration of a cell membrane that the neurotransmitter fits into like a key. If there is a fit, then the cell responds to the neurotransmitter, electrical transmission is allowed to occur, and chemical reactions take place. If there is not a fit, then the cell does not respond.

A psychoactive drug can cause a particular kind of receptor to become more numerous and thereby receive more of its custom neurotransmitters. The same drug can suppress the activity of other kinds of receptors such that they receive less of their neurotransmitters. In such a way, certain brain activities are ramped up while others are damped down.

Another possible way for a psychoactive drug to affect the brain is to block the nerves from taking neurotransmitters out of commission once they have done their job of activating the nerve ending at the receptor site. This keeps more of a particular neurotransmitter swirling around in the space between cells where it can act again and again and again on the receptors on the nerve endings. In nature, it would have acted once and then immediately taken up and stored or metabolized in the cell. Blocking "uptake" causes a tremendous activation of nerve activity such as would never occur normally.

Yet another way for a psychoactive drug to interact with the brain is to partially mimic the natural neurotransmitter, but to cause a distorted effect. For example, dopamine is a naturally occurring neurotransmitter; some drugs fit into the brain's dopamine receptors, but do not act like the body's own dopamine molecules.

The entire system of brain activity could be imagined like a network of high-speed roads regulated by millions of security gates with varying degrees and kinds of traffic getting through. When a psychoactive drug is thrown into the fray, the brain's traffic control is bypassed. The actual situation is not so simplistic. In fact, it is estimated that there are more neurons in the brain than the Milky Way has stars. But this basic model has spawned tremendous growth in the invention of new psychoactive drugs intended to override normal brain mechanisms.

Dr. Candace Pert was the co-developer of the test that detects and measures neurotransmitter receptors in the brain. Dr. Pert's discoveries earned her the title of the mother of *psychoneuroimmunology* (from *psych* "mind" + *neuro* "brain" + *immunology* "the study of the immune system"). However, she was horrified by how her discoveries were used to aggressively promote drug solutions to mental distress. She was even more perturbed by how the emphasis on drugs as miraculous solutions misled the public about the actual damaging effects of the drugs. Dr. Pert was alarmed that the prescribing physicians themselves had little understanding of the derangements in brain biochemistry their drugs were causing. Prescribing doctors ignored the fact that these same neurotransmitters are also found elsewhere in the body. For example, receptors for one such neurotransmitter, *serotonin*, are found on blood cells, in heart muscle, on the uterus, and in the bladder. Most of the body's serotonin receptors are in the intestines. The widespread distribution of serotonin receptors explains of a lot of the adverse physical effects of serotonin drugs. [2]

Serotonin is a neurotransmitter found in the skin of toads in the 1940s. It doesn't just refer to a single substance, but is actually a family of related biochemicals found widely in plants and animals such as in wasp venom, on walnuts, and in the bark of some South American trees.

Therefore, serotonins have many functions and are not just transmitters of nerve impulses in the brain. Serotonins have been found to be mainly responsible for the psychedelic trippy hallucinations of psilocybin (derived from a mushroom) and mescaline (derived from a cactus).

Serotonin activity gets jacked up by LSD (*lysergic acid diethylamide*). LSD was used as a prescription psychiatric drug beginning in 1937 until it was taken off the market in 1966. The world's primary manufacturer was the Swiss company Sandoz Pharmaceuticals who gave it the trade name Delysid. [3] It had three main uses, according to the package insert from Sandoz in 1964:

1. to produce hallucinatory psychosis in mental patients;
2. to experimentally produce psychosis in normal people so as to study mental disorders;
3. for the psychiatrist himself to take so he could experience the world of a mental patient.

It is unclear what the therapeutic effect of LSD was supposed to be. There is no standard medical report of long-term outcomes for patients who were intentionally made to be psychotic by physician-administered LSD. In any case, suicides and permanent insanity in recreational LSD users led to its demise as a medication. However, the LSD link to serotonin was pursued with enthusiasm by drug development researchers in pharmaceutical labs.

Building on the serotonin connection discovered with LSD, the first generation of drugs created to specifically affect brain chemicals included Desyrel and Wellbutrin. These were followed by a second generation that included Prozac, Paxil, and Zoloft. The marketing strategy for these later drugs was to brand them as selective serotonin reuptake inhibitors, or SSRIs, conveying the idea to physicians and patients that these drugs affected only serotonin out of all the many different neurotransmitters ("selective"), and that their single action was to keep serotonin from being taken up by the cell once it had been used ("reuptake inhibitor"). In fact, the drugs affect other neurotransmitters besides serotonin. There are many different subtypes of serotonin receptors and the drug affects them each differently. The SSRI explanation was a mere marketing concept based on an unproven hypothesis with little evidence, but it was used in a very effective campaign to maximize acceptance of the drugs.

The initial patients experimentally treated with these drugs were reported to have some improvement in their depressive symptoms. Building on the hypothesis that mental distress is strictly a biochemical problem, and knowing the drugs affect brain chemistry, the spin fashioned by the marketing departments was to claim that the drugs balanced brain chemistry. This was the 20th century version of the old mystical balancing of humours. It was pretty lame as it did nothing to differentiate these new drugs from any other antidepressant on the market. Therefore, the general concept was morphed into a fictional story of the drugs specifically correcting an imagined serotonin deficiency. The SSRI myth quickly turned into supposed "fact."

The deception inherent in the SSRI moniker is well recognized by anyone who has scratched the surface. Scientists have looked in vain for any consistent science to support the notion of a serotonin deficiency in depressed people. It is now obvious that early researchers did not know exactly what they were measuring when they found serotonin in various plants and animals and in human brain tissue. In 1979, it was discovered that there were at least two distinct subtypes of serotonin. In the 1990s, the number of serotonin types grew to five, and by 2000, seven different serotonin "families" and at least fifteen different subpopulations had been identified. Leading researchers in the serotonin field say that the explosion of discovery of distinct serotonins has caused the scientific nomenclature to be "bewildering." The serotonins are related in that they are made of a base molecule of *tryptophan*. (Tryptophan is a simple amino acid that is a necessary protein to most living systems.) They all have an oxygen-hydrogen group in the 5th position of the base molecule. Beyond that similarity, serotonins vary widely in chemical composition, location of receptors, and the actions they cause.

A particular drug can affect some or all of the serotonins, and in different ways. Trying to track exactly what version of serotonin affects which receptors, and exactly how "has become a nightmare for those involved in identifying or developing site-selective [drugs]" says one experienced drug developer. [4]

The reality is that patients who complain to their doctor of depressive symptoms never have their serotonin levels measured for these two reasons:

1. the level of serotonins in the bloodstream bears no relationship to serotonin levels in the brain;

2. the brain level of serotonins is constantly fluctuating and cannot be directly measured.

It turns out that some serotonin-related brain activities are up-regulated by the drugs and some are down-regulated. Some brain activities are put into hyper-speed and others are suppressed. What this has to do with "reuptake inhibition" is uncertain. Furthermore, drugs in this class directly or indirectly affect several other neurotransmitters besides serotonin. These include the classes of neurotransmitters known as *norepinephrine, dopamine, acetylcholine, GABA,* and others.

There have been hundreds of studies trying to prove the serotonin hypothesis, but none have provided the conclusive evidence drug-makers need. An experiment intentionally lowering the serotonin levels of healthy subjects failed to cause depression. [5] Opposite experiments were also carried out: mood did not improve when huge increases in serotonin levels were caused by direct injection of serotonin into depressed subjects. [6] After a comprehensive review of the extensive medical literature on serotonin, the German Medical Board concluded reports of serotonin deficiency supposedly being responsible for violent suicide attempts were based on flawed scientific methods. [7]

Drug companies are supposed to compile research results and provide the data to the FDA to validate that their drugs are effective. A close look shows that in about half of such studies submitted to the US FDA between 1987 and 1999, the drugs were no more effective in treating depression than placebo. It turns out the studies unfavorable to their drugs were not sent in for publication in medical journals, so they stayed largely out of view to physicians. [8]

Multiple studies dating back to 1981 have repeatedly demonstrated regular exercise alone can improve mood in mild to moderate depression. [9] In one study, people with depression taking Zoloft were compared to depressed patients doing aerobic exercise alone: 60-70% in the exercise group had no signs of depression at the 16-week mark. But persons on antidepressant drugs are not considered cured, only "managed" and their symptoms are expected to recur when they stop the drugs. [10]

In 2005, the *Journal of the American Medical Association* reported on a comprehensive review of nearly 30 years of depression studies and concluded that drug benefits were "minimal to non-existent" for mild to moderate symptoms. In severe depression, the drugs had a 13% advantage over placebo. Usually anything less than 20% is not even considered supportive of further drug development. Even witch doctors average a 20% improvement in their patients. [11]

How do the drug companies get away with manipulating and withholding facts and producing false information by way of marketing strategies? If one reads carefully, drug package inserts, labels, and advertisements contain phrases like "it is presumed" and "the mechanism of action is thought to be" and "scientists believe." These nuances get dropped out of any conversation between the drug sales rep and the doctor, and between the prescribing physician and his or her patient. [12] Read the conflict of interest chapter to discover why these drugs got FDA approval in the first place.

CHAPTER 6

Depression Drugs

All drugs given for depression have an unknown *mechanism of action*: specific biochemical interaction through which a drug substance produces its pharmacological effect. They are classified according to their marketing names. It is beyond the scope of this book to cover all potential adverse drug effects, so we will focus on effects of the most commonly prescribed drugs.

SSRI class

Since the so-called SSRIs affect other brain chemicals besides serotonin and do not only cause inhibition of serotonin reuptake, we cannot accurately call them selective serotonin reuptake inhibitors. These drugs are no more effective for depression than an exercise program, so we cannot accurately call them antidepressants either.

However misleading, the agreed-upon medical naming convention is to call them the SSRI class of drugs. These include brand names: Celexa, Lexapro, Luvox, Paxil, Prozac, Zoloft, Sarafem, Pexeva, Brisdelle, Selfemra, and Raniflux. Other drugs that can affect various aspects of brain serotonin metabolism but are not typically included in the SSRI marketing class include: vilazodone (Viibryd), vortioxetine (Brintellix), buspirone (Buspar), etoperidone (Axiomin, Etonin), and trazodone (Desyrel). They are included here because of having a similar side effect profile.

While they have not been proven to be significantly therapeutic in most people for whom they are prescribed, the SSRI drugs certainly have very well documented side effects. The bulk of the FDA-mandated package insert for an SSRI is dedicated to listing adverse drug effects. Here is a translation in lay language of the generally known adverse effects of these drugs, drawn from the information provided in the package insert for the most commonly known drugs for this class: Prozac, Paxil, and Zoloft. [1]

All antidepressants, including the SSRI class of drugs, carry a prominent *Black Box Warning.* In order to call your doctor's attention to a very serious drug hazard, the FDA requires a warning be at the top of the package insert and surrounded by a bold-font black outline. The Black Box Warning for antidepressants relates that suicidal thinking and suicide attempts (*suicidality*) are more common in children and young adults on antidepressants compared to depressed subjects who take a sugar pill. Studies of suicidality are insufficient in people over 24. What is not mentioned in the warning is the fact that these drugs can also cause suicidality in previously normal people who are not even depressed.

The package inserts relate that there is not enough information to know if SSRI drugs are safe in people with serious illnesses, heart disease, high blood pressure, epilepsy, or liver disease. Older people are more prone to side effects. SSRI drugs should not be used in pregnancy. Life-threatening bleeding may occur in patients also taking blood thinners and/or anti-inflammatory drugs.

In the section on "possible unwanted effects" the drug makers list that SSRI drugs can cause:

anxiety
agitation
panic attacks
insomnia
irritability
hostility
aggressiveness
depression
amnesia
sleeping problems
teeth-grinding
intense emotional ups and downs
apathy
abnormal dreams

- impulsivity
- restlessness
- mania
- paranoia
- hallucinations and delusions
- sexual problems in men and women

The patient and family must be alert to these frequent side effects so they are not mistakenly blamed on "just more mental illness."

The case of Christopher Pittman is a tragic example of SSRI side effects. As a troubled 12-year old, he ran away from his father's home, was picked up by the police, and put in a youth facility. There he was evaluated and deemed to have no mental illness, but prescribed Paxil anyway. Then he was placed under the care of his grandparents. Shortly, he was noted to have new aggressive behavior at school. No one considered this could be an adverse effect of Paxil, even though aggression is listed on the Paxil package insert as mandated by the FDA. Instead of considering toxic medication side effects, the boy was simply switched from Paxil to Zoloft. The Zoloft was prescribed at a relatively high dose of 100mg for his 52", 95-pound frame, then doubled to 200mg after the first week. After just three weeks on Zoloft, under the influence of a drug delirium, and with no prior history of violence, this youngster shot his sleeping grandparents with a .410-gauge shotgun and then set the house on fire. Christopher later said he had auditory hallucinations on the drugs, hearing voices telling him to kill his grandparents. Incredibly, he was tried as an adult. The judge acknowledged there was an element of "involuntary intoxication," yet gave the child a 30-year sentence. This was later shortened to 25 years. [2]

The SSRI class of drugs can also cause dangerously low sodium, which in turn causes headaches, difficulty concentrating, memory problems, confusion, weakness, unsteadiness (may lead to falls), hallucinations, black outs, seizures, coma, stopping breathing, and death.

Weight loss is more common on the SSRI class drugs than increased appetite, especially in children. These drugs can cause seizures and have not been adequately tested in people who already have epilepsy.

Infrequent to rare problems listed by the manufacturers include:

coughing
difficulty breathing
nose bleeds
asthma/bronchitis
sinus infection
menstrual problems
vaginal pain
heavy periods
missed periods
joint pain
uncontrollable movements
muscle cramps
muscle weakness
thirst
fever accompanied by shaking
skin swelling
difficulty swallowing
cavities
burping
heart burn
stomach pain
itch
hives
hair loss
dry skin
rash
sensitive to sun/light
twitching
confusion
dizziness
nerve disorders
migraine
leg cramps
abnormal eye movement
increased saliva
cold clammy skin
pupil dilation
hyperventilation
inability to breathe
coughing up blood
voice loss
life-threatening heart rhythm abnormalities
acne

SSRI drugs can also cause:

muscle pain
nerve problems
back pain
chest pain
increased heart rate
weakness
general discomfort
low sugar levels
low blood counts
eye bleeding
colon inflammation
rectal bleeding/inflammation
stomach ulcers
bulging eyes
growth of breasts in males
bony growths
excessive hair growth
skin discoloration
coma
jerky movements

sensitive hearing
other hearing problems
face swelling
sores in the mouth
black/bloody stools
mouth swelling
hiccup
urgency to urinate
weak muscles
paleness
eye disorders
painful erections in the absence of sexual desire
dilated blood vessels
altered blood platelet function abnormal blood results
other mouth diseases

These drugs can lead to an overload of serotonin resulting in *serotonin syndrome.* Serotonin syndrome is a particular set of bizarre psychic disturbances occurring along with drastic physical signs that can be life-threatening:

agitation
hallucinations
unstable heart rate
unstable blood pressure
very high temperature
abnormal neurologic reflexes
incoordination
nausea
vomiting
diarrhea

Serotonin syndrome can occur when taking a single drug, but is especially likely when more than one drug affecting serotonin is used at the same time. Serotonin syndrome can progress to coma and death.

Coming off of drugs in the SSRI class causes a *discontinuation syndrome* with severe mental and physical effects of drug withdrawal, such as:

mood swings
emotional extremes
agitation
dizziness
tingling
pricking or numbness of the skin
electric shock sensations
anxiety
confusion
headache
sluggishness
severe trouble sleeping

Though not classified as being addictive in that they do not create a craving, there is a definite physical addiction as indicated by the withdrawal symptoms. This has been attributed to the brain having adjusted to the drugs continually keeping serotonin in the synapses between neurons. There is evidence in long-term SSRI users that the brain serotonin receptors are fewer in number and diminished in sensitivity. So when the drug is stopped, the brain does not have the adaptive mechanism it once possessed to keep a normal amount of serotonin around. If withdrawal is attempted, it should be gradual and supervised by a physician. Babies born to mothers on this class of drugs can go into severe drug withdrawal.

Long-term use of SSRIs has been shown to lead to a severe neurologic condition: *tardive dysphoria* (from *tardive* "late" + *dysphoria* "low mood"). Multiple researchers have documented that long-term SSRI users have a loss of frontal lobe function and a loss of ability to think, reason, and make decisions. Children and the elderly are at the highest risk for this effect. [3]

Any mind-altering drug can lead to violent behaviors, but paroxetine (as in Paxil and Brisdelle) is at the top of the list of psychiatric medications most commonly reported to the FDA MedWatch site to cause suicidal and homicidal ideation. [4]

An example of an actual case of violence reported to the FDA can be found on the blog at the Mad in America website:

"This case involves a 16-year-old male from Canada taking Prozac, who experienced the reported drug reaction of 'homicide.' The reporting psychiatrist assessed the homicide, self-injurious behavior, manic symptoms, and worsening of his condition as related to fluoxetine, it drove him over the edge and it contributed to his actions." [5]

Newer SSRI-like drugs

Newer drugs for depression have not been shown to be any more effective than the older drugs, although they do come with catchier names:

Viibrid (vilazodone)

Fetizma (levomilnacipran)

Trintellix (vortioxetine)

They affect multiple neurotransmitters, sometimes in unpredictable ways. All three of these drugs are approved for treating major depression, even though they all carry the Black Box warning about an increased incidence of drug-induced suicidal thoughts and possibly suicide, even in people who were not suicidal before.

Vilazodone (Viibrid) has prominent adverse mental effects including:

suicide	numbness and tingling
serotonin syndrome	abnormal dreams
mania	restlessness
severe withdrawal if it is stopped abruptly	insomnia
headache	fatigue
dizziness	decreased sexual interest
excessive sleepiness	tremor[6]

Physically, Viibrid causes very high rates of diarrhea and nausea, and causes vomiting frequently. It can cause excessive bleeding, especially if taken with anything else that affects blood clotting. Viibrid can cause sudden glaucoma with potentially permanent vision loss and can precipitate seizures. It causes increased appetite and weight gain, ejaculation problems, palpitations, and joint pain. It can cause neurological and breathing problems in newborns of mothers on the drug.

Levomilnacipran (Fetzima) mental effects include:

suicide	tension
serotonin syndrome	aggression
agitation	migraine
anger	numbness and tingling
teeth gnashing	black outs
panic attack	tremors and balance problems[7]

Fetzima carries special warnings for these physical effects:

hypersensitivity (severe allergic reaction)	trouble passing urine
elevated blood pressure	dangerously low sodium
fast heart rate	seizures

abnormal bleeding

increased eye pressure leading to glaucoma and loss of vision

neurological and breathing problems in newborns of mothers on the drug

In addition, Fetzima frequently causes

nausea
vomiting
constipation
excessive sweating
hot flushes
decreased appetite
erectile dysfunction
testicular pain
ejaculation problems[7]

Vortioxetine (Trintellix) can cause:

suicide
mania
serotonin syndrome
dizziness
abnormal dreams

Trintellix causes these physical problems:

nausea
diarrhea
dry mouth
constipation
vomiting
excess gas
weight gain
acute pancreatitis
hypersensitivity (allergy)
abnormal bleeding
sudden increased eye pressure leading to glaucoma and visio loss
low sodium
itching
neurological and breathing problems in newborns of mothers on the drug[8]

SNRI class

Drugs marketed for their effect on both serotonin and the neurotransmitter norepinephrine are categorized as serotonin norepinephrine reuptake inhibitors, or SNRI. These include:

desvenlafaxine (Pristiq)

milnacipran (Ixel, Savella)

duloxetine (Cymbalta)
levomilnacipran (Fetzima)
tofenacin (Elamol, Tofacine)
venlafaxine (Effexor)

Other drugs that have effects primarily on norepinephrine and serotonin include: mianserin (Bolvidon, Norval, Tolvon). Some drugs primarily affect serotonin plus norepinephrine, but they are not in the marketing category of SNRIs. These include mirtazapine (Remeron) and setiptiline (Tecipul). The drug classifications are entirely arbitrary. They open the door for pharmaceutical marketers to suggest that difficult patients can be treated with drugs from multiple classes and can be switched from class to class. The side effect profiles from class to class demonstrate just how similar they all are.

All of the SNRIs can cause all of the adverse events also listed for SSRI class drugs, including withdrawal syndromes and possible tardive dysphoria. Venlafaxine (Effexor) and duloxetine (Cymbalta) are in the top five drugs reported to FDA MedWatch as associated with violence; specifically self-injury, suicidal tendency, or homicidal ideation. [9]

The SNRI poster drug is Effexor—a true brain-scrambler. The Effexor molecule has some structural similarities to the street hallucinogen PCP (phencyclidine, also known as Angel Dust, Supergrass, Boat, Tic Tac, Zoom, Shermans). In fact, some routine urine drug screening tests can turn up positive for PCP in people who are on Effexor. [10]

The list of PCP effects as provided by the US Drug Enforcement Administration (DEA) consistently parallels the list of adverse drug effects on the Effexor package insert, except Effexor's list is much longer. They both affect serotonin, norepinephrine, and dopamine. Like PCP, the SNRIs can cause sedation, drowsiness, stupor (zombie-like state of appearing awake, but not aware of surroundings) lack of energy, and coma. [11] Also like PCP, all of the SNRIs can cause stimulation, including increased heart rate, increased blood pressure, sweating, skin flushing, dizziness, weight loss, excessive salivation, feelings of *euphoria* (high), feelings of strength and invulnerability; and can cause diarrhea, anxiety, agitation, and tremors.

The list of abnormal behaviors caused by Effexor, and the rest of the

SNRIs, is three times as long as the abnormal behavior list for PCP. This list includes: [11]

- amnesia
- confusion *depersonalization* (a sense that one is not themselves)
- disordered thinking
- *apathy* (an immobility induced by hopelessness)
- wildly fluctuating emotions
- hysteria
- hostility
- mania
- psychosis
- suicidal ideas
- feeling drunk
- *delusions* (believing something that cannot be true)
- *illusions* (seeing something that is not there)
- loss of control over impulses
- paranoia
- depression
- hostility

SNRIs can cause *akathisia:* a drug-induced, intense restless anxiety along with physical components of agitation. The word comes from Greek *a* "without" + *kathisis* "sitting." SNRI–induced akathisia makes the user feel like they cannot sit still or sleep, and can trigger a constant state of agitated motion such as pacing and nervous leg and hand movements. Violence can also be a component. In fact, the Effexor label carries a *homicidal ideation* warning. The most notorious of many reports of Effexor-associated violence is the case of Andrea Yates: the Houston-area nurse who methodically drowned her five children in the bathtub, then tucked their bodies into bed before turning herself in to authorities. [12] It wasn't until two years after the tragedy that drug manufacturer Wyeth quietly added homicidal ideation as a rare side effect. The FDA defines rare as occurring in 1 in 1,000 or less. The year of the Yates tragedy, there were over 19 million prescriptions written for Effexor, creating a potential for more than 19,000 homicidal patients living openly and freely within our society. The warning was placed on page 36 of the 47-page package insert in 6-point font. [13]

The Effexor manufacturer received an official Warning Letter from the FDA in 2007 criticizing its ads in professional (doctor) journals for the extended release form of the drug. The FDA said, "The journal ad is misleading because it overstates the efficacy of Effexor XR, makes unsubstantiated superiority claims, in addition to other unsubstantiated claims, and minimizes the risks associated with the use of Effexor XR."[14] The drug maker was obliged to tone down its ad.

Are glossy journal ads really misleading physicians? You betcha!

Didn't they go to medical school to understand this stuff? One wonders.

After four years in college, four years of medical school, a year of internship, and several years of a specialty residency program, reading medical literature is not rocket science. Any doctor should be able to compare drug dosages and schedules, understand the statistical analyses used, and appreciate the many factors that could have influenced or skewed results.

Aren't they capable of interpreting studies themselves? Apparently not!

But it is their responsibility to review the straight facts of any drug they prescribe, instead of relying on the drug company sales reps, glossy ads, or the drug company sponsored medical education seminars to tell them what to think.

Don't prescribing physicians at least unfold and read the package insert? Nope.

Is it too much to ask doctors to take some care in considering if they really want their patients to be subjected to the serious adverse effects of this drug?

Physicians are supposed to do all of that, and in turn, discuss the known adverse effects with the patient so the patient can make an informed decision about whether or not to take the drug. But that almost never occurs.

Consider the case of Dr. Kou Wei Chiu—31-year old Nashville family practice physician—who had been on Effexor. In July of 2007, Dr. Chiu was in Seattle for business, but had forgotten to bring his medication, resulting in him being without it for several days. Of course, the drug distributor's prescribing information provided to physicians warns it can cause personality changes and psychosis and should not be discontinued suddenly. Dr. Chiu was late for his homebound flight, so he used airport payphones to call in bomb threats three times before he was apprehended. He was allowed to travel home (by road) to Tennessee while awaiting trial. He was ultimately given a sentence of 3 years' probation. [15]

These drugs affect so many different neurotransmitters in so many different ways that it is anybody's guess what their major action is. The manufacturer is required to state on the package insert of all drugs given for depression that the mechanism of action (what the drug is doing) is unknown. They all have Black Box Warnings about causing suicidality.

Don't depend on doctors for a thoughtful critique of drug studies. Don't expect doctors to be aware, much less inform you, of all of the Black Box Warnings and potential drug side effects. And especially don't expect doctors to volunteer information on the statistics of how well (or poorly) a drug works, for they are only likely to tell you what the drug ads claimed.

It is your job to be an informed consumer, and your doctor's job to work for you.

1. Ask how the drugs work. They will have to honestly tell you that the mechanisms of action are unknown.

2. Ask about safety. They will have to get the package insert and explain it to you in language you can understand, not medical mumbo-jumbo.

3. Ask about the chances of it working at all. They must tell you the statistics of long term studies in people with your condition who are your age, race, and gender.

4. Ask about viable alternatives to the proposed treatment. Remember they are obligated to answer you honestly and without conflict of interest impacting the answers to your questions.

CHAPTER 7

Sedatives: Anxiety Drugs and Sleeping Pills

Benzodiazepines

Drugs marketed to treat anxiety include the class called *benzodiazepines*, named after their chemical structure. They alter the body's handling of messenger chemicals in the brain. The drug connects to receptors that monitor awareness level, muscle tone, coordination, and memory, and suppresses electrical transmission of nerve impulses in the brain. Benzodiazepine drugs are capable of producing all levels of central nervous system depression from mild sedation to hypnosis and coma. A more descriptive term for this class of drugs is "sedative hypnotics." They all cause sedation. These drugs put the user in a hypnotic state where, even while awake, everyday conversation can have the effect of a hypnotic command. [1]

Physical and psychological dependence occurs with all drugs in the benzodiazepine class. There is some risk of dependence even after relatively short-term use at the usual doses. Therefore, these drugs are classified as controlled substances, meaning that they can only be dispensed in limited amounts and frequency. Stopping the drug suddenly can cause severe withdrawal symptoms. [2]

The classic "benzo" used to be diazepam (Valium and other brands), which is now eclipsed in sales by alprazolam (Xanax and other brands). Other commonly prescribed drugs in the benzo class include Ativan,

Librium, Tranxene, and Serax, but there are nearly a hundred different versions of benzodiazepines.

Any drug in the benzodiazepine class, such as Xanax, can cause:

drowsiness
lack of coordination
fatigue
confusion
weakness
dizziness
blackouts

Xanax and related drugs can cause:

sleepiness
headache
vivid dreams
garbled speech
talkativeness
restlessness
anxiety
mania
false sense of well-being
shakiness
sleep disturbances
nightmares
agitated excitement
hyperactivity
sudden rage reactions
increased muscle spasticity
lightheadedness
abnormal involuntary movements
muscle twitching
fatigue
irritability
inability to think straight
poor memory
depression
nausea
vomiting
diarrhea
increased sweating
fast heart rate
blurred vision

The withdrawal symptoms of Xanax and related drugs come on quickly and rapidly increase. The person feels anxiety and fear, which quickly grows into a sense of panic and grief with a severely low mood. It can progress straight to suicide. During withdrawal, a person suffers extremely unstable emotions and can be prone to sudden outbursts of panic or crying. They start to feel that everything seems "unreal" and they don't feel like themselves, "like in a waking dream." They can get nightmares, become delirious, and experience hallucinations (hearing voices and seeing things that are not there). A person not only feels like they are crazy, but the withdrawal can actually make them go insane.

The person suffering benzodiazepine withdrawal (such as from Xanax) commonly gets a tremor and headache, the heart starts to beat fast, and the person feels "palpitations" or skipped beats. Normal sounds and movements of people or things in the environment easily startle them. They are super-sensitive to touch, get hot and cold sensations and muscle pain. Their increased perception of physical things can be extreme, such as feeling their eyes are pressing into their head, or their teeth are rocking in their gums, or their arms are falling off. They may have trouble doing things with their hands in a coordinated way, and difficulty with swallowing or talking. They feel dizzy and unsteady. All of these mental and physical sensations can convince them that they are experiencing a dread disease like heart attack or stroke. A person in withdrawal can have a seizure and lapse into unconsciousness (coma).

It is very difficult for a person to come off of Xanax or other benzodiazepines without help, monitoring, and calming nutritional support. In summary, taking Xanax—or any drug in the benzodiazepine class—is extremely hazardous. The hell of withdrawal means that, all too often, what gets prescribed for a short term very quickly becomes a long-term addiction. [3]

The stresses of everyday life usually do not require treatment with a drug. This is really good news, for two reasons:

1. Benzodiazepines are addictive after as little as three weeks on the drug.

2. Withdrawal symptoms from benzodiazepines are always worse than what they were initially prescribed for.

For chronic anxiety, drug treatment is also a poor choice because the longer a person is on the drug, the more likely they are to experience multiple adverse drug effects. Furthermore, there are no controlled studies to prove the long term effectiveness of benzodiazepines. For example, studies of Xanax to treat anxiety have lasted only 4 months, and for use in treating panic disorder, it has only been studied for 4 to 10 weeks. [3]

Other sedatives

A related group of drugs are not structurally benzodiazepines, but interact with the benzodiazepine receptors and therefore cause similar effects on the brain. These are usually marketed as sleeping pills, with the most popular being Ambien, Lunesta, and Sonata. Like the benzos, all of these related drugs are classified as controlled substances.

Eszopiclone (Lunesta) is the most representative drug of the sleeping pills. The way these drugs work is not known, but it is clear they alter the brain's normal handling of nerve transmission chemicals, particularly the so-called GABA receptors that monitor wakefulness. They are sedative/hypnotics. These drugs carry a special warning about abnormal thinking and behavior.

Lunesta and related drugs can cause:

Decreased inhibition like out of character aggressiveness and extroversion.

A person may cook and eat food; make phone calls; drive; or have sex without being fully awake, then have no memory of it.

Amnesia and other psychiatric symptoms may occur unpredictably.

Can cause worsening of depression and lead to suicide.

Sleeping pills frequently cause:

anxiety
confusion
depression and hallucinations
dizziness
chest pain
nervousness
migraine headache
increased rate of viral infection especially respiratory infection
dry mouth
stomach upset
nauseas

swelling of hands and feet
increased muscle tone
strange nerve sensations
incoordination
paradoxical insomnia
rapid eye jerking
dizziness
unstable/unbalanced walking
numbness
high feeling
painful perception of physical sensations

vomiting
sleepiness the next day
rash
unpleasant taste
slowed movements
inflammation or paralysis of nerves
stupor
tremor

These drugs may cause:

allergic reaction
skin inflammation
face swelling
fever
bad breath
heat stroke
hernia
weakness
neck rigidity
light sensitivity
high blood pressure
vein inflammation
poor or increased appetite
gall stones
blood in the stool
mouth ulcer
thirst
tongue inflammation
colitis
trouble swallowing
stomach irritation
hepatitis
liver enlargement
liver damage
stomach ulcer
tongue edema
rectal bleeding
anemia
high cholesterol
weight gain
weight loss
dehydration
gout
low potassium
arthritis
bursitis
joint swelling
stiffness
pain
leg cramps
twitching
muscle weakness
acne
hair loss
dermatitis
dry skin
eczema
skin discoloration
sweating
hives
painful red bumps on legs
boils
herpes zoster
abnormal hair
dry or inflamed eyes
ear pain

- swollen lymph nodes
- ringing in the ears
- breast engorgement
- breast cancer
- painful urination
- blood in the urine
- ear infection
- lack of periods
- breast enlargement
- breast pain
- breast milk
- having to pee frequently or loss of bladder control

The drug makers warn that the day after taking Lunesta or related drugs, the person may be impaired and should not do tasks or jobs requiring mental alertness or motor coordination such as driving.

Like benzodiazepines, sleeping pills have the potential to be abused. There is a physical withdrawal that can happen after stopping the drugs, including: anxiety, abnormal dreams, nausea, and upset stomach.

Withdrawal may cause:

- agitation
- apathy
- emotional instability
- hostility
- memory loss
- neurosis
- difficulty concentrating
- abnormal thinking

The patient and their family must be alert and watching for these effects so that the patient is not mistakenly labeled as having a mental illness.

Pregnant women or nursing mothers should not take sleeping pills. Patients with liver disease and the elderly are more sensitive to sedative effects. Depressed people should not take them. Lunesta and related drugs have caused cancer and decreased fertility in both male and female lab rats.

The manufacturer of best-selling Lunesta reports a study showing that it helped people get to sleep only 12 to 15 minutes sooner than people taking a dummy pill. The common drug side effects are a high price to pay for such a slim advantage. [4]

CHAPTER 8

Mood Altering Drugs

When a person has mood shifts or undesirable behaviors that do not fit into any other category, they can always be called *bipolar* or labeled with a *mood disorder.* Bipolar is a relatively recent addition to the psychiatric naming convention. If someone is sluggish in the morning; pepped up after coffee; and then slumps in mid-afternoon, but gets a second wind later in the night, they may well have an underlying thyroid gland deficiency or dis-regulation of hormone output from their adrenal glands. They may be in need of hormones, fish oil supplements, or diet modifications and exercise. However, they are more likely to get medicated for bipolar disorder rather than receive medical tests or lifestyle modification advice.

In European countries, the diagnosis of bipolar is not considered to be valid in people under age 18; they consider ups and downs in this age group to be an aspect of normal childhood. In the US, the fastest growing group of people with a diagnosis of bipolar or mood disorder is youngsters. A study done by researchers at Columbia University found that in 1994/95, only about 1,000 doctor's office visits involved a diagnosis of bipolar in persons under 20; by 2002/03 that number went up to over 1.5 million. Meanwhile, the figure also doubled for adults. [1]

Virtually all persons with this diagnosis are medicated with mood drugs, neuroleptics, or drugs for depression. They are typically on more than one kind of drug or on a cocktail of all three. The so-called "mood regulating" drugs will be addressed in this chapter, with antidepressants and neuroleptics each covered in chapters of their own.

Seizure drugs

Drugs traditionally used to treat epilepsy seizures can cause mild to profound sedation. Even though patients labeled bipolar do not have epilepsy, it is the sedation side effect of epilepsy drugs that was thought to be desirable in patients labeled with a mental disorder. The most common drugs in this category include divalproex (Depakote), valproic acid (Depakine), and valproate (Depacon, Epilim). The adverse effect profiles are similar.

The package insert for Depakote and related drugs carry a Black Box warning mandated by the FDA: all of these drugs increase the risk of suicidal thoughts, suicide attempts, and completed suicides, even in patients who were not suicidal before starting the drug. The warning also indicates these drugs are highly toxic to the liver, and liver injury can progress to life-threatening liver failure. It is necessary for the doctor to monitor liver function tests while a person is on any of these drugs. Potentially fatal inflammation and bleeding into the pancreas can occur. Aside from just affecting the liver or pancreas, drug-induced failure of several internal organs at once can occur. In addition, there is a Black Box warning against using these drugs in the elderly as they can cause dangerously excessive sedation even in usual doses.

Depakote and related drugs can cause malformation of the baby in the womb when taken during pregnancy. The drugs can cause low *platelet* counts (the sticky blood elements that help blood clot); the first sign of this can be bruising, bleeding from the gums, bloody nose, and/or blood in the stool. Can also cause derangements in the blood chemistry, resulting in exposing the brain to such high levels of ammonia that it causes dementia. They can short circuit the brain's normal temperature regulating mechanism, resulting in very low body temperatures, which could cause coma

The most common adverse reactions of seizure drugs include mood swings, despite the fact that this is exactly what the drugs are supposed to be treating.

Other common psychiatric effects include abnormal thinking, amnesia, nervousness, mania, or depression.

The drugs can cause neurologic problems, including:

excessive sleepiness
headaches
blurred vision
double vision
ringing in the ears
imbalance when trying to walk
tremor
rigid muscles.

Depakote and related drugs can cause: [2]

general weakness
nausea
vomiting
stomachache
diarrhea or constipation
acid reflux
poor appetite with weight loss
flu-like illness
infection
bronchitis
sore throat and runny nose
bleeding
bruising
swelling
weight gain
rash
hair loss

Lamotrigine (Lamictal) is another mood drug borrowed from its primary use of suppressing seizures. The way this drug works is not known.

Lamictal frequently causes:

confusion
depression
anxiety
irritability
insomnia
concentration difficulties

Can also cause:

amnesia
abnormal thoughts
abnormal dreams
depression
numbness
abnormally increased sexual desire
abnormal reflexes
irritability
suicidal ideation

The drug maker advises that Lamictal may have to be stopped if any new mental symptoms come up. All antidepressant drugs increase the risk of suicidality in children and young adults, but Lamictal has not been studied enough to see how much it may increase suicidal thinking and actions. If being used for a mental condition, the patient and family should be aware of these mental side effects so they are not mistakenly diagnosed with more mental illness, and only suppressed with yet another drug.

The Black Box warning for Lamictal indicates it can cause a serious and sometimes life threatening rash, especially in children. Sometimes the rash can progress to cause skin shedding and leave disfiguring scars, or even cause death. If a rash is going to happen, it usually occurs in the first two months of treatment, but it can crop up at any time; even after being on the drug for a long time. Lamictal can also cause serious allergic reactions that may first show up with fever and swollen lymph nodes, even without a rash. This can worsen and progress to causing the failure of major bodily organs, and death.

Other unwanted effects of Lamictal can include:

speech problems
dizziness
tremor
unbalanced walking
sleepiness
headache
double vision
blurred vision
abnormal jerking of eyes
swelling of the face
bleeding
dry mouth
bad breath
nausea
vomiting

nausea
diarrhea
bleeding from the rectum
fever
swollen lymph nodes
itchy skin
infection
bronchitis
shortness of breath
flu-like illness
sinus infection
inflamed and runny nose
bloody nose
anxiety
insomnia

inability to coordinate movements
stomach pain
acid reflux
peptic ulcer
constipation
loss of appetite
weight loss
joint pain
weakness
chest pain
neck pain
abnormally painful periods
accidental injury

Lamictal can cause abnormalities in blood counts, with extremely low counts of infection fighting cells, low red blood cells causing anemia, and low platelets leading to inability to normally clot the blood.

Lamictal can cause drowsiness, sleepiness, and general depression of brain functions.

When Lamictal is suddenly stopped, this can cause seizures to suddenly re-appear, or in patients treated for something besides seizures, can cause seizures to occur even if the patient never had seizures before.

Lamictal has not been adequately studied in human pregnancy, but is known to interfere with the body's ability to make B vitamin folate. Folate deficiency in pregnancy can lead to deformed babies. It also passes into breast milk, so should not be taken by nursing mothers.

Lamictal binds to areas of the body that are colored, such as the iris of the eye and pigmented skin, but how this affects health is not known.

The drug stays in the body longer in females and non-Caucasian patients.

In patients with liver disease, Lamictal may cause heart electrical irregularities. [3]

Lamictal is approved for use in adults with a bipolar diagnosis, but studies claiming to prove it works for mental conditions are under fire as being highly flawed. Use of Lamictal for mood disorders in children has not been adequately studied to see if it is safe or if it works. The drug maker is required to submit at least two studies to the FDA showing the drug's effectiveness. GlaxoSmithKline submitted one study that barely showed an advantage for Lamictal in the initial phase of bipolar. They scrambled to come up with a second study, and funded several that failed to show any effectiveness of their drug; they didn't publish those or submit them to the FDA. Finally, GSK funded a study that compared Lamictal to lithium (the original drug for this condition) and Lamictal supposedly performed better at delaying the time to relapse of bipolar depression. The flaw in this study design was that of all the people put on either drug, only those that responded continued on the drug and were reported on when the study was published. All patients did eventually relapse. It was on the strength of this kind of junk science that Lamictal gained approval by the FDA. [4]

Carbamazepine (Tegretol) is another seizure drug sometimes prescribed to treat mood and bipolar diagnoses. A related drug is oxcarbazepine (Trileptal), which has a similar side effect profile. Like all seizure medications, these drugs carry a warning about suicidality, with Tegretol causing twice the risk of suicidal thinking and behaviors even in people who had no suicidality to begin with. The package insert for Tegretol includes a Black Box warning about serious skin reactions (skin looks as if it were burned and just peels away) that can be life threatening, which are more likely to occur in people with Asian heritage or in those carrying a specific gene type. Another of the Black Box warnings is for a type of profound anemia that can wipe out all blood cell lines (red, white, and platelets), or the drug may decimate only the white blood cells, resulting in inability to fight infection.

Tegretol and related drugs can cause severe psychiatric disturbances, including confusion, visual hallucinations, depression with agitation, excessive talkativeness, and drinking excess water to the point where sodium is so low that it causes brain swelling. It can also cause the brain to make excess hormone such that too much salt is lost through urination, and the brain cannot function with such low sodium. Seizure and coma may result.

Tegretol and related drugs directly affect the brain and nerves where they can cause:

- dizziness
- drowsiness
- inflammation of the tongue
- aching muscles and joints

trouble with coordination
headache
fatigue
blurred vision
double vision
abnormal jerking of the eyeballs
difficulty talking
loss of control of movements
painful nerves
numbness
ringing in the ears
extreme sensitivity to sound
nausea
vomiting
stomach upset and pain
diarrhea
constipation
loss of appetite
muscle cramps
non-specific fever and chills
calcium loss, leading to soft bones
congestive heart failure
swelling
worsen high blood pressure
cause abnormally low blood pressure
worsen heart disease
blood clots and abnormal heart rhythms leading to death
liver inflammation and failure
inflammation of the pancreas
shortness of breath
pneumonia
increased urination
trouble passing urine
kidney failure
dry mouth and throat

It is also one of many psychiatric drugs that can cause *neuroleptic malignant syndrome* where the body loses its temperature regulating ability, resulting in extreme fevers (106 degrees Fahrenheit) that literally cook the brain. This causes seizures, coma, and can be deadly.

Paralysis and other symptoms of stroke have been reported in people on Tegretol.

There have been reports of increased eye pressure (leading to glaucoma) as well as abnormalities of the lenses of the eyes.

In addition to the life-threatening skin reactions, these drugs can cause several other skin reactions ranging from red rashes to coloration of the skin to hives, pustules, spots, bruising, fingernails and toenails falling off, and loss of hair or excess hair growth all over the body.

In men, it can cause an inability to get an erection, abnormal sperm development, and shrinkage of the testicles.

When any epilepsy drug is suddenly stopped it can cause a seizure to occur even in people who never had epilepsy. [5]

Other seizure medications such as gabapentin (Neurontin) and topiramate (Topamax) are not FDA approved for bipolar, but are often used *off-label*. Off-label means the FDA has not found the drug either safe or effective for these conditions. It is not illegal for the doctor to prescribe in this way, but it requires that the patient understand the off-label nature, and the implications that its use is strictly experimental.

Gabapentin (Neurontin) has an unknown mechanism of action, but is similar in structure to the natural body chemical GABA, which overall suppresses or depresses nerve firing and causes sedation.

Neurontin frequently causes:

disturbing mental changes, including hostility, confusion, depression, and anxiety
memory loss
abnormal thoughts
abnormal dreams
hallucinations
feeling high
feeling doped-up
personality disorder
increased or decreased sexual desire
mania
antisocial personality
suicidal thoughts
suicide
paranoia

The patient and family must be alert to these potential effects so the patient is not mistakenly labeled as having a mental illness.

Neurontin use has been associated with breast cancer and brain cancer.

This drug frequently causes:

a general weak feeling
tiredness
face swelling
joint pain
dizziness
hyperactive movements

high blood pressure
poor appetite
gas
gum inflammation
bruising

numbness and tingling
abnormal reflexes
pneumonia
vision problems

Neurontin can also cause:

weight gain
back pain
swelling
dilation of vessels
heartburn
nausea
dry mouth and throat
constipation
dental problems
increased appetite
low white blood cell count
muscle pain
broken bones
coordination problems with unsteady movements or staggering
involuntary eyeball movements
uncontrollable muscle movements or shaking
nervousness
speech problems
runny nose
sore throat
coughing
itchy skin
inability to have sex (impotence)
muscle spasms

excessive thirst
inflamed stomach/intestines
drooling
hemorrhoids
bloody stools
uncontrolled bowel movements
liver enlargement
anemia with a drop in all blood counts
arthritis and other joint problems
tendon inflammation
fainting
muscle tone deformities
paralysis of one side of the body and face
partial loss of consciousness
impaired motor skills
swellings filled with blood
apathy
nosebleed
difficulty breathing
hair loss
dry skin
eczema
increased sweating
excessive hair growth

tingling
tickling
itching
burning
bleeding into the brain
allergy symptoms
weight loss
chills
low blood pressure
chest pain
fast heart rhythm
migraine
inflammation of tongue
gum bleeding
ringing in ears
oily skin
herpes
blood in urine
painful urination
painful menstruation
sexual abnormalities
cataracts
inflammation of eyes
dry eyes
eye pain
eye bleeding
eye twitching
earache
hearing loss
loss of taste

Rarely, Neurontin can cause:

heart failure
brain damage
slow heart beat
inflammation of heart
swallowing pain
burping
pancreas, esophagus, and colon inflammation
stomach ulcer
blisters in mouth
tooth discoloration
chapped lips
bleeding lips
hernia
blood in vomit
rectal bleeding
hyperthyroid
hypothyroid
antisocial personality
suicide
hyperventilation
hiccups
laryngitis
runny nose
snoring
lung swelling
shingles
skin discoloration
pimple outbreaks
sensitivity to light
ulcers
lumps on legs/arms
oily scalp
skin peeling and skin death
vaginal discharge

low levels of female hormones
ovarian failure
swollen testicles
increase in white blood cell count
increased bleeding time
osteoporosis
rib inflammation
osteoporosis
permanent muscle contraction
nerve damage or nerve death
uncontrollable facial movements
brain diseases
personality disorder
increased sexual desire
mania
kidney pain/kidney stones
genital itching
kidney failure
inability to urinate
high amounts of protein/sugar in urine
breast pain
testicle pain
noise sensitivity
eye focusing problems
watery eyes
glaucoma
tear duct blocking
blindness
other degenerative eye problems
smell dysfunction

Side effects that have been reported after the drug was approved but not in drug company studies include:

ringing in the ears
stomach pain
hepatitis
jaundice
liver failure
low sodium in the blood
kidney failure
acne
hair loss
painful purple rash preceding top layer of skin death and shedding
abnormal breast growth in men

Neurontin is not approved for use in pregnancy. It passes through breast milk to the baby.

Manufacturer studies show even more psychiatric drug effects occur in children 12 and under. Children also can get viral infection, fever, nausea, vomiting, and sleepwalking from Neurontin. [6]

Topiramate (Topamax) has the same suicide warning as all of the antiepileptic drugs. It can cause depression and mood problems even though it is often used to treat the same; the family should be aware these could be drug-induced so as not to have them mistaken for just more symptoms of underlying mental illness.

This drug can cause:

difficulty in thinking clearly
change in personality
anxiety
confusion
tiredness and fatigue but also insomnia
memory problems
language difficulties
speech problems
tingling sensations
difficulty walking
sudden buildup of fluid pressure in the eye leading to glaucoma and vision loss
vision loss even without fluid buildup
kidney stones
infection
weight loss
poor strength
diarrhea
headache
dizziness
slowness
difficulty with concentration and attention

Topamax can override the body's normal regulatory mechanisms by causing decreased sweating and extremely high fever or extremely low body temperature. It can derange blood chemistry by creating an acid condition in the blood or high ammonia levels leading to dementia and coma.

Used during pregnancy, it can cause deformities in the baby. [7]

Lithium

Lithium is a highly toxic mineral found in the earth's crust. It is in the same chemical family as sodium, but has profoundly different effects. Lithium is sold as Lithobid, Eskalith, and other brand names. Like all of the psychotropic medications, the mechanism of action is not known.

Lithium has a very narrow window between a dose that causes calming and a dose that causes toxicity—therapeutic level is 0.6 mEq/L and immediate toxicity occurs when the levels are over 1.5 mEq/L. This makes it an especially hazardous drug and it is necessary to keep track of drug levels by blood tests, as well as frequently checking for organ damage.

Lithium's mental effects can include nervousness and depression despite the fact that this is what it is supposed to treat. Other mental effects can include:

confusion
low energy
extreme sluggishness, which can progress to coma
slurred speech
difficulty swallowing
dizziness
a sensation of spinning
muscle twitching
trembling of the hands
loss of bowel control
seizures

Neurologic drug effects include *pseudotumor cerebri,* a condition of too much fluid pressure on the brain. It results in headaches, loss of urine control, and imbalance when trying to walk.

Lithium commonly causes low thyroid. It interferes with the production, activation, and use of *thyroid hormone* (a substance that normally regulates metabolism). Some estimates are that up to half of people on long-term lithium eventually develop low thyroid.

Lithium can also disrupt the *parathyroid glands* (4 parathyroid glands sit on the corners of the thyroid gland in the neck) and result in dangerously abnormal calcium levels.

Lithium is highly toxic to the kidneys, being directly poisonous to kidney tissues. Lithium-affected kidneys cannot concentrate urine normally, and cannot get rid of acid efficiently. At least one in every ten people on lithium get kidney damage, but studies of people taking lithium over many years suggest this number goes up to 70%. Lithium damage to kidneys is irreversible. [8,9]

Lithium can cause:

blurred vision
loss of appetite
sensitivity to cold
seizures

weight gain	abnormal heart beat (slow, fast, or irregular palpitations)
muscle weakness	heart throbbing or pounding
nausea	increased thirst
vomiting	increased frequency and urgency to pass urine
pain	skin rash
coldness	stomach bloating
blue coloration of fingers or toes	

Less common but potentially severe effects of lithium can include: [10]

abnormal heart electrical signals	dry mouth
abnormally low blood pressure	high blood sugar
disturbance of any of the senses affecting the limbs	inflammation of hair follicles
blind spots	involuntary eye movements
blurred vision	swollen ankles or feet

All of these drugs can cause the exact moodiness they are supposed to treat, which shows up on the package inserts as "emotional lability." When a mood-altering drug is said to be working, most of what is being described is sedation. Subdued people are considered improved, even if that was not the improvement they were looking for. These drugs have the potential to cause much worse mental derangements than a flighty mood, especially with long-term use and in combination with other psychotropic drugs.

CHAPTER 9

NEUROLEPTIC DRUGS

Neuroleptic drugs (from *neuro* "brain" + *leptic* "to take hold or seize") used to be reserved only for institutionalized psychotics. They are also referred to as chemical straightjackets, major tranquilizers, or antipsychotics. In the past twenty years, the use of neuroleptic drugs has been massively popularized so that now they are given for nearly anything one can find in the *Diagnostic and Statistical Manual.* Many of these uses for neuroleptics are off-label (beyond what the FDA has approved). [1]

The earliest versions of neuroleptic drugs were derived from work done on insecticides and anti-worming agents, which paralyzed the nervous system of bugs very effectively. The key to affecting the nervous system was to block the brain's receptors for dopamine, although we now know these drugs affect many other neurotransmitters besides dopamine.

The drugs Thorazine, Stelazine, Mellaril, Haldol, and others eventually got a bad rap when it became evident that nearly all patients on long term treatment ended up with drug-induced movement disorders. These included *dystonia*, which is continuous spasm and cramping of muscles. A more severe drug-induced movement disorder is *tardive dyskinesia* (*tardive* "delayed"; *dys* "abnormal" +*kinesia* "movement"). Uncontrollable jerky limb movements, facial grimacing, tongue contortions, and lip smacking characterize tardive dyskinesia—the bizarre movements can identify a long-term psychiatric patient from a block away. Tardive dyskinesia can develop after short-term use, but is more likely to happen as treatment continues. Tragically, it is usually permanent, even after stopping the drug.

Many people taking neuroleptic drugs also eventually develop a version of Parkinson's disease, with an expressionless face, tremor, freezing episodes, muscle rigidity, bent and shuffling walk, and slowness of thought and movement.

Another severe drug effect is *akathisia*, the condition of profound inner agitation mirrored by extreme physical restlessness. Akathisia has been demonstrated to lead to the patient acting out violence, oftentimes severe. Although akathisia was first associated with neuroleptic drugs, it is now known to occur with almost any psychiatric drug.

Yet another consequence initially thought to be unique to neuroleptic drugs is the *neuroleptic malignant syndrome* (NMS), although NMS is now seen with many other classes of psychiatric drugs. The syndrome is a life-threatening neurological disorder consisting of muscle rigidity, high fever, autonomic instability, and cognitive changes such as delirium. The high fever and seizures of NMS have a 50% fatality rate if not quickly recognized and treated. The brain cell killing effect of neuroleptic drugs is so well recognized that these drugs have been investigated as chemotherapy for brain cancers. [2]

In the 1980s, a second generation of neuroleptic drugs was introduced. They affect dopamine and serotonin. The mechanism of action of neuroleptic drugs has not been established. Neuroleptics primarily affect dopamine and serotonin, but also have effects on the neurotransmitters norepinephrine, acetylcholine, and histamine in the brain. The main drug effect, which is interpreted as improved behavior, is sedation. Simply put, these drugs act like a chemical restraint.

The dopamine effects were toned down to a certain extent, so that advertising promised the awful movement disorders (NMS, akathisia, and Parkinson's) would be rare. Such was not the case. All of the problems with the first generation drugs are in fact listed as potential adverse effects of the second-generation drugs. The drugs include:

risperidone (Risperdal)
olanzapine (Zyprexa)
clozapine (Clozaril)
quetiapine (Seroquel)
aripiprazole (Abilify)
ziprasidone (Geodon)

They are being prescribed to alter mood; for autism, mania, depression, bipolar, anxiety, post-partum blues; and everything in between.

The brain-damaging effects of these drugs are obvious in their side effect profile, but actual brain scans tell the story biochemistry cannot. The loss of brain tissue shown in MRI scans of schizophrenic patients is more related to the patient's duration of neuroleptic (antipsychotic) drug use than the severity of their illness, age, alcohol use, or any other variable. In other words, the loss of brain tissue is directly related only to neuroleptic drug use. [3]

The side effects are nearly identical from drug to drug in this class, so the best-selling Risperdal will be used here as the example drug.

Like all of the neuroleptics, the package insert warns about suicidality.

Despite the fact that neuroleptic drugs were initially recommended to the most psychotic of mental patients, the drugs themselves cause a person to become psychotic. A patient on neuroleptics can develop full-blown psychosis with delusions, hallucinations, and disordered thinking even if they never had psychosis before taking the drug. These drugs can cause psychosis as effectively as LSD.

Other psychiatric effects include depression, difficulties in thinking straight, insomnia, sleepiness, restlessness and agitation, anxiety, confusion, and increased disturbing dreams.

The patient and family must be alert to potential side effects so they are not mistakenly blamed on "just more mental illness" as happened in the tragic story of Andrea Yates. Mrs. Yates was a mother of five, including a newborn, when her husband concluded she had post-partum depression based on an internet questionnaire. Her treatment included increasing doses of a neuroleptic drug (Haldol), despite having no psychotic symptoms initially. Exactly as warned on the manufacturer's package insert, she gradually developed disordered thinking. Instead of tapering down and off the offending drug at that point, the doctor prescribed ever more medication. Eventually, her doctor documented she was psychotic from the Haldol. He then ignored the drug maker's recommendation and stopped the drug suddenly, at the same time doubling the dose of her other psychiatric drug, Effexor, as described in Chapter 5. It was under these circumstances that she drowned each of her five children, tucked their bodies into bed, and called 911 to turn herself in. In addition to sudden withdrawal from Haldol and excessive dosing with Effexor, she suffered from *polypharmacy*, wherein drug interactions sharply increase the risk of adverse effects.

Neuroleptic drugs can cause slowness in body movements, stroke, permanent uncontrolled body movements, Parkinson's-like tremors and stiffness, and swallowing difficulties leading to pneumonia.

Risperdal and related drugs can cause:

a sudden drop in blood pressure when standing	dizziness
seizures	diarrhea
black outs	constipation
extremely high fever	increased saliva
extremely low body temperature	infertility
low white blood cell count (impairing the ability to fight infections)	sore throat
muscle stiffness	dry mouth
indigestion	hunger
nausea	stomach pain
blurred vision	loss of control of urine
muscle aches	rash
rapid heartbeat and possibly fatal heart irregularity	blood-clotting problems leading to massive bruising [4]

All of the second-generation neuroleptic drugs can cause dystonia, tardive dyskinesia, Neuroleptic Malignant Syndrome (NMS), and drug-induced Parkinson's.

The majority of patients will develop some type of movement disorder in the course of their treatment. In a study reported on the Risperdal package insert, the incidence of a movement disorder after only 8 weeks on the drug ranged from 17% at the lowest dose to 35% at the highest dose. Of course, most patients taking neuroleptic drugs are on them for months and years, and the cumulative incidence of movement disorders continues to increase. [4]

The treatment for drug-induced movement disorders is to switch the patient to a different neuroleptic drug. This takes advantage of the fact that each of the neuroleptic drugs affect the dopamine receptors in slightly different ways. The idea is that the first drug has deranged the brain's neurotransmitter receptors to an extreme degree; a different neuroleptic drug bumps that first drug off their positions on the dopamine receptors and has slightly different effects. For some reason that is poorly understood, this is just enough to alleviate the abnormal movements. Switching to another neuroleptic drug may work entirely or partially, but movement disorders often recur while on the new drug. In any case, the patient is stuck on neuroleptic drugs for a lifetime. When NMS fails to respond to a switch in drugs, electroshock is used.

The drug effects on neurotransmitter receptors makes these drugs hazardous at any age, but especially so for children whose brains are still forming crucial connections.

The second-generation neuroleptic drugs frequently cause weight gain, high cholesterol, high blood sugar, and diabetes. Abnormally high blood sugar can come on very rapidly and result in death from diabetic coma before diabetes is even diagnosed.

These drugs can cause increase in the brain hormone prolactin, which comes from the pituitary gland in the brain. Most of the major neuroleptic drugs have been linked to growth of pituitary tumors, with risperidone being the most common one reported. Increased prolactin causes breast enlargement, which may lead to increased risk of breast cancer in men and women; breast milk, even in men; and also causes impotence. Neuroleptic drugs in high doses can cause tumors in lab rats, particularly breast cancers. The high prolactin also causes thinning of the bones, and people on neuroleptic drugs have more than two and half times the incidence of hip fractures. [5]

Neuroleptic drugs are not approved for treatment of dementia, and in fact have a Black Box warning against this. Over a dozen studies have demonstrated that elderly patients with dementia on neuroleptic drugs have more than one and a half times the death rate compared to patients taking a dummy pill. Despite the warning, these drugs are commonly used in nursing homes because it is easier to handle sedated patients who are bedridden in a drug stupor than to attend to alert, complaining patients.

There is limited testing of the safety of neuroleptic drugs in pregnancy, but some newborns of medicated mothers have had immediate muscle stiffness, breathing difficulty, or seizures. Many of the neuroleptic drugs pass into breast milk and can cause movement disorders in babies.

The FDA has approved risperidone to suppress the explosive and aggressive behaviors in children with autism; it is simply "working" as a chemical restraint. The neuroleptic drugs do not alter core behaviors of autism and suppression wears off when the drug is stopped. Some children are put on more than one neuroleptic drug for diagnoses such as the mania of bipolar or schizophrenia, and they have a vacant appearance: they have little spontaneous speech, look aged, movements are robot-like, and emotions are blunted.

Any neuroleptic drug can have a withdrawal syndrome. The deadliest withdrawal symptom is psychosis, which can result in violence or suicide. Symptoms leading up to psychosis are common, including tremendous anxiety, sleeplessness, nausea, stiffness, pain, headaches, mood changes, and concentration difficulties. A person wishing to come off these drugs must work closely with a doctor who will not mistakenly interpret the withdrawal symptoms as "just more underlying mental illness." Neuroleptic drugs should never be stopped suddenly as this can cause psychosis even in someone who never had psychosis before being medicated.

Signs of addiction include drug-seeking behaviors such as stealing to satisfy the craving for the drug. Addictive behaviors have been reported with all of the neuroleptic drugs, but are most common with Seroquel, Risperdal, Zyprexa, Abilify, Haldol, and Geodon.

The newest safety warnings on aripiprazole and related drugs describe a particular psychosis that emerges. While pathological gambling had already been recognized, there are now mandatory warnings about binge eating, binge shopping, and uncontrollable urges to have sex. [6]

Newer neuroleptic drugs

Newer drugs in this class have not been shown to be any more effective than the older medications. They include:

cariprazine (Vraylar)
brexpiprazola (Rexulti)
They both carry Black Box warnings about increasing the rate of suicide in younger people, and for hastening death in the elderly. These drugs promote premature death in the elderly from all causes, but especially pneumonia and heart failure. They cause an increase incidence of strokes. They cause Neuroleptic Malignant Syndrome, which can be deadly; it is described in full earlier in this chapter.

These drugs cause:

heart failure
respiratory failure
stroke
increase falls
tardive dyskinesia
high blood sugar
diabetes
high cholesterol
weight gain
low white blood counts,
low blood pressure
black outs
seizures
body temperature not controlled
swallowing problems leading to choking
fast heart rate
constipation
stomach pain
dry mouth
nausea, vomiting
elevated liver enzymes
high blood pressure

Mental effects include:

- suicide
- akathisia
- tremor and balance problems
- headache
- dizziness
- agitation
- insomnia
- restlessness
- anxiety
- impair judgment
- scrambled thinking
- poor motor skills
- sleepiness
- fatigue[7]

Coming soon to a prescriber near you are the brave new world class of digital drugs. These smart pills consist of your drug embedded in an edible sensor. The patient wears a patch that senses the readouts via Bluetooth, detecting if the pill has been taken or not.

According to advertising from the makers of digital aripiprazole, this technology is needed because "Taking a medicine as prescribed can be hardship, especially with a mental health disorder." In reality, it will police medication compliance and likely be used to force mental treatment. [8]

Neuroleptic drugs have also been implicated in promoting addiction to commonly abused street drugs. Ironically, the neuroleptics are being investigated for use in assisting with the treatment of addiction, which appears to be a case of substituting one brain damaging effect for another. [9]

CHAPTER 10

Stimulant Drugs

Amphetamines

Amphetamine, dextroamphetamine, methamphetamine, and their various combinations are all known as amphetamines. In fact, their chemical properties and actions are so similar that even experienced users have difficulty knowing which drug they have taken. They are similar in structure and action to cocaine. Amphetamines, cocaine, and related drugs interact with the brain's receptors for dopamine, among many other neurotransmitters. When sold on the playground or on the street, these very same amphetamines go by the names speed, kiddy cocaine, poor man's cocaine, meth, crystal meth, ice, glass, or yaba. Drugs in this class include Concerta, Ritalin, Adderall, Dexedrin, Daytrana, Metadate, Quillivant, Vyvanase, Desoxsyn, and Focalin. Amphetamines are controlled substances because of their addiction and abuse potential.

Amphetamines and related drugs are categorized as stimulants, although any psychotropic drug (including the sedatives) can have stimulant properties—earlier chapters described anxiety, restlessness, akathisia, agitation, and violence caused by many different classes of drugs not categorized as stimulants. An everyday example is alcohol, which acts as a stimulant in low doses (the happy talkative drunk), acts as a depressant in higher doses (the drinker blacks out), and can even cause coma in situations of profound intoxication.

It is not clear how the idea originated to give stimulant drugs to children who were considered hyperactive; it is certainly not logical on the face of it. However, like alcohol, amphetamines can have sedative effects in high doses. The dose used in children is on the high end, relative to their body weight. In other words, a usual dosage given to cause wakefulness in adults is likely to have sedative effects in children. Schoolchildren can usually identify which of their classmates are on Ritalin or Adderall because they are slow in movement and dull in their responses, and may even have a glazed-over look. Their classmates call them zombies, and researchers have recently confirmed that stimulant drugs cause an imbalance in dopamine regulation, producing this zombie effect. [1]

Like other psychiatric drugs, the mechanism of action is not known—it's the sedative effect that is desired in treating unwanted behaviors in children.

The example drug to best describe the adverse effects of all stimulants is Adderall. Adderall and related drugs all carry a warning about being highly addictive. It is a fact that any child on these drugs for more than a few days can suffer addiction: when the drug is stopped, he or she will have physical and mental symptoms of withdrawal.

Withdrawal symptoms include:

- depression
- anxiety
- fatigue
- paranoia
- aggression
- intense cravings, including a craving for cocaine [2]

The package insert carries prominent FDA-mandated warnings that the drug can cause the following serious mental derangements:

- psychotic behavior
- aggression
- violent behavior
- anxiety
- confusion
- paranoia
- insomnia
- hallucinations
- mood disturbances
- delusions
- personality changes

The patient and family must be alert to these drug effects so they are not mistakenly blamed on "just more mental illness."

The true impact of the potential for these drugs to cause suicide and even homicide is not communicated when they are merely mentioned on a package insert in tiny 6-point font, or as numbers in columns of charts. Instead, it is reading about what happened to real people that drives home the risks.

It is incredibly difficult to get what should be publically-available reports of drug effects. Some documentation has been obtained by the persistence of researcher Andrew Thibault, who relentlessly pressures the FDA for the information by using Freedom of Information petitions and even lawsuits.

On his informative blog at the Mad in America website, Thibault posts this example:

Re: Vyvanse

"Case # 10213468, USA, 2014: A 3-month-old female infant was left alone with a babysitter's 10-year-old daughter. Lisdexamfetamine was prescribed to the 10-year-old daughter of the babysitter; the 10-year old girl had ADHD, ODD, and attachment disorder. The infant sustained various injuries. The autopsy reported the cause of death was 'asphyxia and suffocation,' as the result of 'homicide.' Additionally, the infant's blood contained traces of amphetamine (lisdexamfetamine)." [3]

Stimulant drugs frequently cause agitation, even though that is what they are supposed to be treating. Ironically, the package insert states Adderall (and related drugs) are not safe in patients with agitation, but those are precisely the youngsters who get put on these drugs.

These drugs frequently cause:

anxiety	emotional mood swings
nervousness	depression
irritability	insomnia or excessive sleepiness, or both

Amphetamines have not been adequately tested for how well they work beyond 3 weeks in children or beyond 4 weeks in adults. Typically, a child is prescribed a stimulant drug for the 9-month school year or all year round, despite the lack of information on long-term safety and effectiveness.

Amphetamines and related stimulant drugs can cause brain damage similar to what is seen in Alzheimer's disease, stroke, and epilepsy. These drugs can cause seizures in children who never had them before, can worsen seizures in epilepsy patients, cause new onset of tics, or worsen existing tics.

Amphetamines can cause heart muscle damage leading to heart failure. Anyone with known heart abnormalities should not take this drug, although most of the reports of sudden death have occurred in youngsters without any pre-existing heart abnormality. Sudden death, stroke, and heart attack have occurred in children and adults on usual doses of prescription stimulants.

Long-term use stunts growth and causes weight loss in children. Vision problems and, rarely, blindness can occur.

Amphetamines can cause:

light-headedness
tremors
slurred speech
headaches
dizziness
decreased sex drive
impotence
painful menstruation
heart palpitations
chest pain
high blood pressure
nausea
sun sensitivity
vomiting
diarrhea
constipation
acid stomach
belly pain
no appetite
weight loss
dry mouth
"meth mouth" with teeth falling out
infection
fever
rash

People on amphetamines have a higher risk of accidental injury.

Babies born to mothers dependent on amphetamines are more likely to be premature and have low birth weight. Newborns often have to be treated in the intensive care unit for drug withdrawal. Amphetamines cross into breast milk and should not be used by nursing mothers.

Amphetamines are not supposed to be prescribed for people with advanced hardening of the arteries, heart disease, high blood pressure, high thyroid, or glaucoma. Stimulants cannot safely be prescribed to anyone who ever abused drugs.

Non-amphetamine Stimulants

Strattera (atomoxetine) is a stimulant drug classified along with amphetamines in European countries, but not classified that way in the US. Because it is not classified as a controlled substance in the US, it is much easier to prescribe than amphetamines and is not closely tracked by the US Drug Enforcement Administration.

Strattera can cause sudden death in children and adults who have no prior heart disease. In the US, Strattera is classified as a selective inhibitor of the reuptake of norepinephrine, which is a brain chemical that acts much like adrenaline. In fact, the drug is not so selective: Strattera also causes an increase in the neurotransmitters dopamine, acetylcholine, and histamine in several areas of the brain.

Like all psychiatric drugs given to children, the package insert for Strattera carries an FDA-mandated Black Box Warning about increased suicidality in children and young adults. The package insert has prominent warnings about the potential of the drug to cause aggression and hostility, and to provoke mania.

Strattera can cause delusions and hallucinations in children and adults who don't have any prior history of mental illness of any kind. Other mental effects of Strattera include:

feeling jittery
nervousness
abnormal dreams
insomnia

anxiety or depression, or both	blackouts
mood swings	severe nervous scratching strong enough to leave marks

Neurological effects of Strattera include tremor, tics, numbness, fatigue, irritability, headache and dizziness. [4]

Strattera can cause:

chest pain	sudden heart death
high blood pressure	increased sweating
rapid heart beat (palpitations)	coldness or hot flushes
worsen existing heart disease	skin rash

Strattera causes liver injury and liver failure, with some deaths; although some affected patients narrowly avoid death by getting a liver transplant.

Strattera causes stomach pain, nausea, vomiting, decreased appetite, weight loss, constipation, dry mouth, blurry vision, eye inflammation, dry eye, difficulty getting an erection, premature ejaculation, menstruation irregularities, decreased sex drive in men and women, and difficulty passing urine.

Animal studies with Strattera have shown it causes severe birth defects, and pups of drugged and nursing mothers had decreased survival rates.

CHAPTER 11

Psychiatric Treatments Causing Direct Brain Damage

A growing number of people are rejecting biochemical psychiatric treatments because of their dangerous and potentially long-lasting effects on personality, brain chemistry, and the nervous system. At the same time, there is a rise in the use of direct physical treatments.

The earliest evidence of direct physical treatment consists of 40 skulls with bore holes found at an archeological site in France dated around 6500 BC. Evidence of *trepanning* (named after the tool used to cut the skull) has also been found in Peru, Guatemala, and Mexico. Trepanning was used for some brain disorders, such as head injury and epilepsy, and for psychiatric purposes from the time of Hippocrates through the Renaissance period. Written records reveal it was considered that some mysterious thing in the head needed to be destroyed or released in order to bring about a halt to unacceptable behaviors—not too different from modern theories.

This chapter features electroshock (ECT) and deep brain stimulation (DBS) physical treatment methods.

Electroshock

The modern era of direct physical attack on the brain for psychiatric purposes started with electroshock (ECT) in the 1930s. Electrodes are applied to the head and an electrical surge is sent through the attached wires of sufficient power to overcome the resistance of the skull and brain tissue. The orderly electrical patterns of nerve transmissions are overridden and a chaotic seizure pattern results.

Early enthusiasts of electroshock were candid about its effects and admitted brain damage was necessary for the "cure." They counted side effects as therapeutic and were bluntly honest about consequences. Devastation of memory and reduced intelligence were touted as the cure for mental illness. In other words, they won't remember what was bothering them and will be too dull to care.

The mechanism of ECT is best described in the words of shock doctors themselves. Prominent American electroshock psychiatrist Dr. Abraham Myerson said in 1942:

"I think the disturbance in memory is probably an integral part of the recovery process. I think it may be true that these people have for the time being at any rate more intelligence than they can handle and that the reduction of intelligence is an important factor in the curative process. I say this without cynicism. The fact is that some of the very best cures that one gets are in those individuals whom one reduces almost to amentia." [1] (Amentia: *a* "without" + *mentia* "thinking ability")

A year later, Dr. Myerson reported, "The mechanism of improvement and recovery [with electric shock] seems to be to knock out the brain and reduce the higher activities, to impair the memory, and thus the newer acquisition of the mind, namely, the pathological state, is forgotten." [2] Myerson considered ECT effective when it caused the person to forget what they were depressed about in the first place.

Other leading shock doctors were just as straightforward with their goals. Dr. Kennedy and Dr. Anchel wrote in 1948:

"We started by inducing two to four grand mal convulsions [major seizures] daily until the desired degree of regression was reached.... We considered a patient had regressed sufficiently when he wet and soiled, or acted and talked like a child of four.... Sometimes the confusion passes rapidly and patients act as if they had awakened from dreaming; their minds seem like clean slates upon which we can write." [3]

The theories of exactly how electroshock worked were wide ranging and included physical explanations such as destruction of presumably abnormal brain tissues, shaking up the circulation, causing spasm of capillaries, magically eliminating diseased nerve cells, and beneficially decreasing brain function overall. Other theories focused on the emotional reactions. For example, the experience supposedly simulated death and then rebirth; shock caused fear, which was therapeutic; it made the patient helpless and dependent on the doctor, who could then act as a mother figure; it destroyed survival instincts and coerced dependence on outside figures; it satisfied the patient's craving of punishment for his sins; persons in a vegetative state were thought to be more adjustable than highly intelligent persons. Electroshock effectively replaced insanity with imbecility.

More theories of how electroshock "works" can be found in the article "Fifty Shock Therapy Theories," by Hirsch L. Gordon, published November 1948 in the *Military Surgeon.* [4]

Forty years later, leading electroshock psychiatrists were describing it in essentially the same terms:

"After a few sessions of ECT the symptoms are those of moderate cerebral contusion [brain injury], and further enthusiastic use of ECT may result in the patient functioning at a subhuman level. Electroconvulsive therapy in effect may be defined as a controlled type of brain damage produced by electrical means.... In all cases the ECT 'response' is due to the concussion-type, or more serious, effect of ECT. The patient 'forgets' his symptoms because the brain damage destroys memory traces in the brain, and the patient has to pay for this by a reduction in mental capacity of varying degree." [5]

By the 1990s, the practice of electroshock still did not have scientific support.

"The treatment [ECT] is admittedly mysterious. One of my colleagues,

Dr. Stuart Yudofsky, once likened it to kicking the television set when the picture is fuzzy. We still haven't the slightest clue why it works." [6]

Author John Horgan toured New York's State Psychiatric Institute as a guest of leading ECT advocate Harold Sackeim, who arranged to let Horgan observe two patients undergoing ECT. Horgan wrote:

"Sackeim compared shock therapy to stepping on a car's gas pedal when an idling engine is revving too fast. 'We're triggering a seizure in order to get the brain to stop a seizure.' This explanation is 'probably the predominant theory right now,' Sackeim said. 'God knows if it's true.'" [7]

Today's theories are of a more technical nature. We hear about neurotransmitters and brain waves, which are in fact identical to changes seen after concussion and blunt head trauma. The brain-damaging effects of electroshock are very well documented.

The ECT machine itself is still categorized by the FDA as a Class III device, meaning insufficient information exists on its safety or effectiveness. In 2012, the Government Accounting Office mandated that the FDA undertake a comprehensive review of medical evidence about ECT. The FDA failed to carry out the mandate and instead selected a few favorable articles to review. These were mostly opinion pieces, not objective scientific studies. The FDA then compounded their negligence by ignoring unfavorable things reported in articles that also praised ECT. The FDA committee blamed the difficulty in evaluating ECT on psychiatrists tending to label any adverse effects as if they were just more of the patient's mental illness. In their executive summary draft, the FDA stated:

"Because ECT is used to treat psychiatric conditions, it is often difficult to distinguish between primary symptomatology and treatment-caused (or exacerbated) effects." [8]

This statement equating ECT effects as just more mental illness was used by the FDA to repeatedly explain how the medical literature was insufficient to address ECT-induced mania and homicidal behavior; ECT-related severe personality changes; post-ECT severe anxiety, fear, and panic; ECT-induced coma; temporary and permanent neurologic damage after ECT, including tremors, muscle twitching, spasms, paralysis, seizures, and lack of muscle control; and ECT-associated nightmares, vision changes, hearing problems, and urinary symptoms.

When seeking to evaluate why increased use of illicit drugs occurs after ECT treatment, the FDA conjured up a similar explanation for not being able to sort it all out:

"Given the increased co-morbidity [concurrent conditions] of psychiatric illness and substance abuse, it is difficult to determine the cause of increased substance use associated with ECT." [8]

Regarding ECT-associated suicide, the FDA cited a study finding that suicides were 42% more likely in the ECT era than in the antidepressant era. [9] The FDA also admitted ECT is definitely associated with a general decrease in the quality of life and more so-called "general functional disability," which includes difficulties attending to activities of daily living and inability to work.

The FDA found ECT-associated body pain to be relatively common. Although the FDA report states pain is "time-limited," this is contradicted by mention of the need to use medication for prolonged pain after ECT. The FDA concluded breathing and heart and blood vessel complications of treatment are among the most frequent causes of significant sickness and death associated with ECT. These include prolonged spells of not breathing, fluid leaking into the airspaces of the lungs, high blood pressure, low blood pressure, abnormal heart rhythms, stroke, and low blood flow to the heart muscle (heart attack).

The FDA report says, "The primary type of retrograde memory affected [by ECT] is autobiographical memory." This type of memory includes such essentials as knowledge of one's own identity, childhood memories, family memories, learning experiences, and work and travel history. They cite a review estimating memory loss is experienced by 29% to 79% of ECT patients, but ignore other reports of up to 99%.

FDA admits three studies show definite brain cell loss due to electroshock and mentions "*neuroproliferation*" (growth of new brain cells) as a possible good effect of ECT. What the FDA report did not mention is the abundance of studies considering such brain cell growth as no more than a response to injury—in fact, post-ECT nerve growth activity is exactly what is seen during recovery from other forms of brain injury. Unfortunately, new brain cells do not integrate into existing brain structure in a normal pattern. After an electric shock, brain cells exhibit persistently abnormal conduction of electricity. [10, 11] This is explained by the finding that connections at the ends of such new brain cells have a deranged structure and are positioned along the nerve in atypical locations compared to normal brain cells. [12]

Medical studies have established ECT shortens life due to increased death from any cause. The largest study ever conducted involved 3,288 patients in Monroe County, New York. Patients were found to have significantly increased death rates from all causes compared to non-ECT treated depressed subjects. [13] Another study of patients who received in-hospital ECT showed they had survival rates of 73% at one year, compared to 96% of depressed patients who did not get ECT still alive at the end of the first year. 54% of the ECT patients were still alive at two years, compared to 91% of depressed but not shocked patients. Barely half (51%) of ECT recipients were still alive at three years, compared to 75% of depressed patients who were not shocked. [14]

The first three years of mandated recording of death within 14 days of ECT in the state of Texas yielded reports of 21 deaths: more than half were cardiovascular, including massive heart attacks and strokes; 14% due to respiratory deaths; and about a third were suicides. Many of these deaths occurred after the patient had left the hospital and, therefore, the role of ECT was not necessarily ever recorded as a possible contributing factor. [15]

In modern day electroshock, the patient is given a sedative, put under general anesthesia to assure unconsciousness during the shock, and given a paralyzing drug to suppress the muscle jerking normally seen with a seizure. So it all looks entirely humane, but the death rates and the immediate and long lasting memory deficits and other mental effects are the same.

While you can find a few patients who claim to be grateful they underwent ECT, even they often admit to long lasting adverse effects. For the final words on shock, here are some statements from people who have experienced it.

Judy Garland returned to the set after finishing a series of 33 electroshock treatments, but recalled later:

"I couldn't learn anything. I couldn't retain anything; I was just up there making strange noises. Here I was in the middle of a million-dollar property, with a million-dollar wardrobe, with a million eyes on me, and I was in a complete daze. I knew it, and everyone around me knew it." [16]

Author Earnest Hemingway said this after undergoing 20 horrific rounds of shock treatments at the Mayo Clinic:

"Well, what is the sense of ruining my head and erasing my memory, which is my capital, and putting me out of business? It was a brilliant cure but we lost the patient. It's a bum turn, Hotch, terrible."

Hemingway committed suicide by shotgun shortly thereafter. [17]

Electroshock survivor Anne Donahue said:

"Human memory seems to me to be one of the most precious aspects of our personality, since our memories are so critical to who we are and how we see ourselves and others. The memories of our past give us an understanding of where we fit in the world. I have experienced more than a 'cognitive deficit.' I have lost a part of myself." [18]

Deep Brain Stimulation

Deep Brain Stimulation, or DBS, is another way of attacking the brain to treat mental issues. Like other misguided psychiatric concepts, DBS is based on a little bit of science and a whole lot of theory. DBS was initially FDA-approved for use in treating the physical brain disease Parkinson's and related movement disorders. It has since been granted approval for use in obsessive-compulsive disorders under the Humanitarian Device Exemption. This exemption means that mental patients can get DBS even though it has not been tested and proven to be safe and effective for them. This is bizarre, since major adverse effects of DBS in Parkinson's patients is mental derangement and fantastically increased suicide rates. [19]

Let's look at how DBS "works." A hole is bored into the skull. A wire, usually two pronged with each end having several electrically-active pods, is poked through normal brain tissue to get at one of many brain areas affected by Parkinson's disease. The patient is awake, but lightly sedated during this stage of the procedure. The wire is dragged around the area and periodically (randomly) the doctor (or a technician from the device company) causes it to go live with an electrical charge. Meanwhile, the patient is checked for how the mini electric shocks affect movement, such as ability to speak, move their arms and legs, and tap their fingers. The patient is also tested for numbness of various body parts. By this method, the doctor decides where the wire should be implanted. Attached extension wires are burrowed under the skin in the neck and chest. The wire in the brain soon lodges into place by scar tissue buildup in the normal healing process. The patient returns for a second surgery to place a combination battery pack and programming chip in the chest, which is attached to the extension wires.

Over the course of the next few weeks, the programming is progressively tweaked—not a very scientific process considering that there are *29,000 possible settings to experiment with.* As the programming is varied, the patient experiences changes in body control and tremor.

Doctors, scientists, and engineers employed by the manufacturer of the device have not figured out the actual mechanism of action of DBS treatment. One theory is that the small amount of heat created by each electrical charge has an effect on the brain messenger chemicals put out by the wrongly firing brain cells. Another theory is that electricity continuously pumped into the brain acts like repeated little "jump-starts" to overcome abnormal nerve impulses. The bottom line is that they still don't know how it works for Parkinson's, and even less is known about how it is supposed to function in overcoming objectionable mental and behavioral issues.

The device was FDA approved because in the majority of cases it reduces or eliminates tremors in Parkinson's patients. This allows some patients to reduce their dopamine medications, which gives partial relief from drug side effects like dyskinesia. DBS has a less reliable effect on the stiffness component of Parkinson's disease and is much less successful in helping Parkinson's patients with their ability to walk, balance, or their tendency to fall, and can make these worse.

Aside from wire breakage and infection, the three major unwanted effects in Parkinson's patients are memory loss, speech problems, and mental decline. Sometimes DBS can actually make Parkinson's worse. Speech can be severely affected, even in patients who had normally flowing speech before surgery. Many studies have shown the treatment does not improve the general sense of well-being in the patient. [20] Even patients who have easier movement do not consistently report their overall quality of life is any better. [21]

Immediately after the device is turned on, or later as a result of changes in programming, the brain stimulation may cause the patient to weep uncontrollably, laugh without feeling happy, yawn repeatedly, or feel inexplicably fearful or anxious. A study reported in the *Journal of the American Medical Association* described DBS patients unpredictably dropping suddenly into apparent deep sleep. [22] The family may report the patient slipping into dangerously low moods, having memory problems, and quickly becoming unable to make everyday decisions. [23]

Anyone with a degenerative neurological disease such as Parkinson's could be understandably depressed and anxious. But large studies like one done at the Veteran's Administration Hospital in San Francisco have shown that deep brain stimulation can make Parkinson patients totally apathetic, lacking emotions and feeling. [24, 25] This results in a fantastically increased incidence of suicide. Doctors from Johns Hopkins did a review of ten years' worth of DBS side effects in Parkinson's patients, and reported the most concerning problems were wire breakage, brain infection, depression, mania, and a high rate of suicide. Parkinson's patients with DBS have *10 times the rate of suicide* compared to patients with usual medication treatment—that's completed suicides. The rate of attempted suicides is *20 times increased.* Studies done by the National Institutes of Health show that DBS patients have anywhere from *13 to 37 times* the suicide rate of elderly without Parkinson's. [26] Thus, it is incredible that DBS is being put to use when mental conditions are the primary concern.

Mental derangement is such a common problem that most centers doing deep brain implants insist Parkinson's patients participate in so-called "multi-disciplinary treatment."[27] This means that before and after surgery, the patient is tested, evaluated, and treated by psychiatrists. The psychiatric evaluation done before surgery may find the patient is already such a high suicide risk that they will not be allowed to get DBS. Other patients may get psychiatric drugs before and after surgery. Any psychiatric symptoms are dealt with by trying to suppress them with medication.

The bottom line is that Parkinson's patients with mental symptoms from deep brain stimulation become lifelong psychiatric patients. As a treatment for this *bona fide* neurologic disorder, DBS actually creates psychiatric patients.

As learned in previous chapters, psychiatric medications do not reverse or cure anything—they just make the symptoms less distressing for family and caregivers. In these patients, any reduction in movement side effects (from Parkinson's drugs) is traded for mental side effects of the DBS itself, and/or the side effects of psychiatric drugs. [28]

DBS is now being done experimentally for depression, bipolar disorder, and a number of other psychiatric conditions. Where to place the wires is a guessing game. The fact is that no one has ever identified any specific anatomic location in the brain that is abnormal in persons labeled with primary mental conditions. The only exception is the structural and biochemical abnormalities consequent to long term treatment, not found in untreated subjects.

Electroshock and long acting psychiatric medication is already routinely being court-ordered, and it is expected that the implanted DBS device will be the next such forced treatment.

Remember that Frankenstein was the name of the doctor, not the emotionally confused and intellectually challenged monster he irresponsibly created.

CHAPTER 12

Psychiatric Drugs Used for Physical Medical Conditions

Drugs for Weight Loss

The history of weight loss drugs is long and shady, with a predictable recurring theme. A miracle drug is announced, hard sell advertising follows, millions take it, and predictable side effects occur (oftentimes deadly). Then, the FDA, who approved it in the first place, holds hearings to review the evidence of toxicity. Finally, it is banned or the drug maker is pressured to "voluntarily" withdraw it from the market. Lawsuits quietly get settled and drug makers walk off with tidy profits. [1]

Suprenza (phentermine) is a drug with a chemical structure similar to amphetamines. It affects many brain neurotransmitters, particularly various serotonins. When phentermine was combined with fenfluramine it became known as FenPhen. It was the best-selling diet pill in history until it was taken off the market for causing deadly heart valve damage. Phentermine alone is still on the market as a drug for weight loss and for depression; in addition to Suprenza, phentermine is marketed under the names Adipex-P, Fastin, Ionamin, or Zantryl.

These drugs can cause a rush of euphoria, then in the same person, also cause sudden very low mood.

Can also cause:

tremor
agitation
weird dreams
insomnia
anxiety
restlessness
depression
weakness
psychosis with delusions and hallucinations
impotence
decreased interest in sex

Due to the addictive nature of amphetamines, phentermine is a controlled substance. [2]

Qysmia is a combination weight loss drug consisting of phentermine and topiramate; it has the combined adverse effects of these two drugs. It is also a controlled substance due to the high potential for addiction to phentermine. Qysmia can cause suicidal thinking and suicide, even in people who had no mental problems before taking it.

Qysmia can cause: [3]

euphoria
mania
psychosis with delusions and hallucinations
agitation
headache
dizziness
difficulty paying attention
poor concentration
memory loss
word finding difficulties
insomnia
depression
anxiety
fatigue
irritability
numbness and tingling
tremor
impotence
lack of sex drive

Contrave is a combination weight loss drug consisting of naltrexone plus bupropion. Naltrexone reacts to the brain's opioid receptors, and because of this, it is used to treat drug addiction, although it does cause some mind-altering effects of its own. Bupropion is a drug usually marketed for depression and it interacts with multiple neurotransmitters. Each drug independently can cause suicidal thinking and suicide even in people who didn't have any mental problems before.

Contrave frequently causes insomnia.

It commonly causes mind-altering effects, including:

abnormal dreams
agitation
anxiety
nervousness
difficulty concentrating
depression

Contrave can cause: [4]

depression
euphoric mood
delirium
decreased sexual interest
brain vessel rupture
convulsions
inattention
distortion of taste
difficulty thinking
migraine
stroke
numbness and tingling
fatigue
headaches

Belviq (locaserin) mainly affects brain serotonin. Like the SSRI class of drugs, Belviq can cause suicide even in people who had no mental issues before taking it. A person taking Belviq can experience *serotonin syndrome* consisting of bizarre psychic disturbances occurring along with drastic physical symptoms which can be life-threatening. These include:

agitation
hallucinations
unstable heart rate
unstable blood pressure
very high temperature
abnormal neurologic reflexes
incoordination
nausea
vomiting
diarrhea

Serotonin syndrome can rapidly progress to coma and death.

People coming off of Belviq can experience a *discontinuation syndrome* with severe mental and physical effects of drug withdrawal such as:

mood swings
emotional extremes
agitation
dizziness
tingling
electric shock sensations
anxiety
confusion
headache
sluggishness

pricking or numbness of the skin
severe trouble sleeping

Belviq can cause *neuroleptic malignant syndrome* with extremely high fever, muscle rigidity, seizures, and brain injury.

Belviq can cause dissociation, in which normally related thoughts and ideas are disconnected from each other; there is a mental and emotional disconnect that leads to irrational behavior. Can also cause: [5]

euphoria
hallucination
depression
anxiety
stress
mood changes
inattention
memory loss
sleepiness
insomnia
confusion
fatigue

Psychoactive Drugs for Restless Legs

All of the drugs prescribed for restless legs syndrome (RLS) have profound psychotropic effects. RLS was practically unheard of twenty years ago, but the drug makers have poured millions into popularizing the diagnosis. RLS drugs that mainly affect dopamine also double as treatments for Parkinson's disease.

Pramipexole (Mirapex) commonly causes hallucinations. The package insert carries an FDA-mandated warning about sudden sleep attacks. Patients are also warned about drug-induced intense urges and loss of impulse control for gambling, spending money, engaging in sexual activity, and binge eating.

Other mental effects include:

amnesia
confusion
sleepiness
weird dreams
dizziness
impotence
lack of appetite
low energy

Mirapex can cause *akathisia*: extreme motor restlessness accompanied by a profound inner tension leading to violence. Withdrawal can cause neuroleptic malignant syndrome with high fevers, muscle rigidity, coma, and death. [6]

The warnings for ropinirole (Requip) are the same, but the package insert gives an additional warning about drug-induced psychotic behavior. This can include paranoid ideas, delusions, hallucinations, disorientation, aggressiveness, agitation, and delirium. [7]

Levodopa (Sinemet and other brand names) converts into dopamine in the body, is the main treatment for Parkinson's disease, and is used in treating RLS. Sinemet and related drugs can cause loss of impulse control and psychotic episodes, including delusions, hallucinations, and paranoid ideas.

Can cause: [8]

confusion
agitation
dizziness
sleepiness
nightmares
insomnia
headache
depression
suicidal tendencies
dementia

Another psychoactive drug used for RLS, bromocriptine (Parlodel, Cycloset), affects dopamine and can cause psychosis with hallucinations and delusions, confusion, agitation, insomnia, hyper sexuality, headache, fatigue, drowsiness and sudden sleep attacks, and dizziness. [9] Likewise, rotigotine (Neupro) for RLS causes sudden sleep attacks, hallucinations, psychotic behavior, loss of impulse control, compulsive behaviors (spending, gambling, sex), and nightmares. [10]

Sedatives are also used for RLS. Example drugs are Klonopin (clonazepam), Xanax (alprazolam), and Restoril (temazepam). These drugs are in the benzodiazepine class (see chapter 7) and mainly affect the GABA receptors that monitor wakefulness, thus they have sedative effects. The overall effect of benzodiazepines is to suppress electrical transmission of nerve impulses in the brain. Benzodiazepines have been given to Sea World's killer whales and are routinely used in animal rescue facilities. [11] They tame aggressive animals and put them into a hypnotic trance—they have the same effect in humans. Klonopin connects to brain receptors that monitor awareness level, muscle tone, coordination, and memory. Benzodiazepine drugs are capable of producing all levels of central nervous system depression from mild sedation to hypnosis and coma.

Benzodiazepines are highly addictive and increase the risk of suicide. They commonly cause:

depression	agitation
amnesia (memory loss)	nervousness
hysterical behavior	hostility
psychosis	anxiety
excitability	insomnia
irritability	nightmares
aggressive behavior	vivid dreams

These drugs weaken the ability to think, to make judgments, and to react and move the body.

Suddenly stopping a benzodiazepine can cause seizures, even in people who did not have seizures before. The withdrawal symptoms prominently include anxiety and fear. This quickly grows into a sense of panic and grief-like severely low mood. It can progress straight to suicide. During withdrawal, a person suffers extremely unstable emotions, making them prone to sudden outbursts of panic and/or crying. The person starts to feel that everything is "unreal" and they are not themselves, "like a waking dream." They can have nightmares, hallucinations (hearing voices and seeing things that are not there), and become delirious. A person not only feels like they are crazy, but the withdrawal can actually make them go insane. He or she commonly gets a tremor and headache; their heart starts to beat fast and they feel "palpitations" or skipped beats. Normal sounds and movements of people or things in their environment easily startle them. They are super-sensitive to touch, get hot and cold sensations and muscle pain. Their increased perception of physical things can be extreme, such as feeling the eyes are pressing into their head, or teeth rocking in their gums, or their arm is falling off. They may have trouble doing things with their hands in a coordinated way, and difficulty with swallowing or talking. They feel dizzy and unsteady. All of these mental and physical sensations can convince them they are experiencing a dread disease, heart attack, or stroke. They can get a seizure and lapse into unconsciousness (coma). [12]

Psychiatric Drugs for Other Physical Conditions

Sarafem is fluoxetine, also known as Prozac, but repackaged and advertised for pre-menstrual syndrome. Sarafem can cause suicide in people who had no prior mental problems. It can cause anxiety, agitation, panic attacks, insomnia, irritability, hostility, aggressiveness, impulsivity, restlessness, mania, depression, amnesia, sleeping problems, teeth-grinding, intense emotional ups and downs, apathy, abnormal dreams, paranoia, hallucinations and delusions, and sexual problems in men and women. Sarafem can cause serotonin syndrome, discontinuation syndrome, and neuroleptic malignant syndrome as described for the SSRI drugs. [13]

Lotronex (alosetron) is a drug given to slow the movement of stool through the colon, and is marketed to people with irritable bowel syndrome. It achieves this effect by interacting with the serotonin receptors lining the bowel; these are the same kind of serotonin receptors found in the brain and the drug is active in both locations. Lotronex can cause:

- anxiety
- depression
- sexual dysfunction
- sudden sleep attacks
- memory problems
- tremors
- sedation
- strange dreams
- difficulty thinking
- disturbances of sense of taste
- balance problems
- confusion
- fatigue
- decreased ability to experience feeling

Any of the adverse effects of an SSRI drug (chapter 6) could potentially occur with Lotronex. [14]

Psychoactive Drugs Prescribed for Headaches

Psychiatric drugs are commonly prescribed for tension headaches, hangover headaches, sinus headaches, dental headaches, ice cream headaches, cluster headaches, medication overuse headaches, caffeine withdrawal headaches, and just plain headaches. There is no conclusive evidence that these headaches have anything to do with altered brain biochemistry or deranged receptors for neurotransmitters, and response to the drugs is generally poor. The sad irony is that every single psychiatric drug prescribed for headaches frequently causes headaches, and withdrawal headaches are common when the drugs are stopped.

Sufferers of non-migraine headaches are often prescribed any one of the drugs usually given for depression, even though the person is not depressed. All such drugs carry a Black Box warning about causing suicidality even in people who were not suicidal or depressed before taking the drugs. Alternately or in combination, headache patients may be prescribed any of the benzodiazepine drugs such as Xanax, or offered sleeping pills like Lunesta, or may be pushed to take so-called mood regulators like Neurontin. Often, the psychiatric drug prescription is chronic, which is especially dangerous for addictive drugs like Xanax, wherein even a three-week course can result in addiction. Accidental overdose is more likely when benzodiazepines are prescribed along with narcotic pain medications. [15]

Headache patients can experience withdrawal symptoms after taking any of the drugs affecting serotonin. In addition, users of the SSRI drugs can experience serotonin syndrome: agitation, hallucinations, unstable heart rate, unstable blood pressure, very high temperature, abnormal neurologic reflexes, incoordination, nausea, vomiting and diarrhea. Rarely, serotonin syndrome can progress to coma and death.

It is especially important to be informed about the potential adverse effects of psychiatric drugs prescribed for medical conditions as the prominent mental effects they cause can be entirely unexpected to the unsuspecting patient. See chapter 6 for a full discussion of side effects, Black Box warning labels, and withdrawal symptoms of SSRI drugs.

The migraine type of headache has been successfully treated with the triptan class of drugs such as sumatriptan (Imitrex) and others. Triptan drugs work by activating a specific serotonin receptor type, which is very unlike the depression drugs that affect multiple serotonins and other brain neurotransmitters. This particular kind of serotonin receptor is on the brain blood vessels, and when activated, it causes the vessels to constrict, opposing the dilating effect of a migraine. However, this is also the source of the drug's most deadly potential side effects: stroke and heart attack. Unlike the psychiatric drugs that more generally affect various serotonins, the mental side effects of triptans are infrequent to rare. [16]

Ergot alkaloids are a class of drugs only rarely used for migraines anymore due to their severe effects and tendency to poison the patient. Ergots are extracted from fungi, which grow on grasses and grains. One group of derivatives is used for migraines, while another derivative is lysergic acid, or LSD. The ergot alkaloids for migraines, such as Sansert, Cafergot, or DHE-45, work by powerfully constricting blood vessels. They can do this so effectively that they may cause stroke or gangrene. The major potential mental effect of ergot alkaloids is drug dependence and addiction. [17]

Psychiatric Drugs Given to Treat Pain

Narcotics are readily prescribed for acute and long-term pain. They can be prescribed alone or in combination with acetaminophen (such as Tylenol #3, Vicodin, Norco) or with ibuprofen. The drugs include codeine and its various forms (dihydrocodeine, hydrocodone, and oxycodone); morphine and its various forms (oxymorphine, oxycodone, hydromorphone, and fentanyl); and meperidine (Demerol). Narcotics always cause drowsiness, mental clouding, weakness, and impairment of mental and physical performance. They can cause anxiety, fear, and mood changes. The main mental effect is addiction, which can even occur after short-term use. 70% of prescribed drugs involved in deadly overdoses are narcotic painkillers, and the remaining 30% are benzodiazepines, most of which are accidental. [18]

Prescription narcotic use in women can cause a newborn to go into life threatening withdrawal shortly after birth. Access to prescription pain medications in the home is a key factor in drug abuse by teenagers. Soldiers and veterans are more likely than others to be on long-term prescriptions for narcotic painkillers, and overuse of prescription painkillers after a work-related injury is becoming an epidemic in workers comp systems. This all adds up to more narcotics being prescribed and abused at every strata of society, with prescription drug addiction now a major problem in all age groups. [19]

Non-narcotic medications for pain also deliver heavy mental effects. The main non-narcotics are gabapentin (Neurontin) and gabapentin enacarbil (Horizant). It is not known how gabapentin works. It is similar in structure to the natural body chemical GABA, which overall suppresses or depresses nerve firing. Neurontin frequently causes disturbing mental changes including hostility, confusion, depression, and anxiety.

Other less frequent mental effects include:

memory loss
abnormal thoughts
abnormal dreams
sleepwalking
hallucinations
paranoia
feeling high
doped-up feeling
personality disorder
increased or decreased sexual desire
mania
antisocial personality
suicidal thoughts
suicide

The patient and family must be alert to these effects so the patients are not mistakenly labeled as having a mental illness. [20]

Drug overdoses now kill more people in the United States than car crashes. Overdose deaths involving prescription opioids have quadrupled since 1999, and so have legal sales of these prescription drugs. Each day more than 1000 people are treated in emergency rooms for misuse of their opiates to get high. In 2014, almost 2 million Americans abused or were dependent on prescription opioids. [21]

In early 2016, there were big news headlines about the FDA "toughening" the warning labels for opioids. But the new warnings are no big deal. In the Warning section meant for doctors, the label now says that immediate-release opioid preparations "should be reserved for pain severe enough to require opioid treatment and for which alternative treatment options are inadequate or not tolerated." [22]

This is really just advice to prescribing doctors, and totally nonbinding—it is not against the law to ignore it. It is highly unlikely to result in any change in the massive inappropriate over-prescribing. There were no dose thresholds or maximum amounts given.

Lyrica (pregabalin) is given for fatigue and nerve pain. It is chemically related to the body's own neurotransmitter, GABA, but the drug has an unknown mechanism of action. Lyrica can be a drug of abuse because of its weird mental effect, and can become addictive.

Frequently causes:

neurologic and mental problems including "depersonalization" (a feeling that nothing is real and you aren't yourself)

- dizziness
- sleepiness
- anxiety
- increased muscle tone
- increased sensitivity
- poor sexual drive
- jerking eye movements
- tingling
- drunk feeling
- muscle twitching

Lyrica also frequently causes body pains, even though it is FDA-approved to treat fibromyalgia. Some of the side effects occurring in people without a previous diagnosis of fibromyalgia are identical to fibromyalgia symptoms.

Lyrica may also cause:

- memory problems including amnesia
- depression
- confusion
- nervousness
- tremor
- insomnia
- hangover effect
- drug dependence
- swelling in the brain
- lack of orgasm

hallucinations
euphoria (false feeling of intense well-being)
slowed or abnormal thinking
difficulty concentrating
language problems
impotence
psychotic behavior
suicidal thinking
suicide attempts

The patient and family must be alert to these effects so the patient is not mistakenly labeled as having a mental illness.

It is not known how this drug acts on the nerves or how it may change brain chemistry when given long term.

When Lyrica is stopped, there can be a withdrawal syndrome consisting of insomnia, nausea, headache, and diarrhea.

It also causes headaches, stupor, and loss of bladder control.

Lyrica has not been proven safe in children or in pregnancy, and it is not known if it passes through breast milk. [23]

Another drug given for pain that affects brain neurotransmitters is clonidine, sold as Catapres, Kapvay, or Nexiclon XR. Clonidine can cause mental depression; hallucinations (hearing things and seeing things that aren't real); numbness; insomnia, vivid dreams or nightmares; restlessness; anxiety; agitation; delirium, mental depression, nervousness, and other behavioral changes; irritability, other behavioral changes, and drowsiness.

Clonidine causes withdrawal syndrome with nervousness, agitation, headache, tremor, and confusion accompanied or followed by a rapid rise in blood pressure, which can lead to stroke. [24]

Quit Smoking Drugs

No drug prescribed for smokers makes a person quit smoking. For that, a person needs to put down the cigarettes and make changes to enable themselves to stop. Using mind-altering drugs comes with great risks in the short term, including suicide and violence. In the long term, they could make a lifelong psychiatric patient out of the person.

Some drugs affect too many neurotransmitters to be conveniently classified. Bupropion is marketed as Wellbutrin for depression and as Zyban for smoking cessation. It affects norepinephrine, dopamine, and nicotinic acetylcholine receptors in unknown ways. Bupropion is also among the top drugs most frequently reported to FDA MedWatch for violence—a category including self-harm and suicidal and homicidal ideation.

In studies the drug maker (Glaxo) paid for to test their drug, bupropion (Zyban), anywhere from 27% to 49% of Zyban users initially quit smoking cigarettes. However, in those same studies, 17% to 23% of subjects taking a dummy pill (placebo) also quit smoking. The more significant finding was what happened six months and one year down the road. After six months, only 19% of Zyban users were still not smoking. At 12 months, there was no difference between those who used Zyban to quit and those who were only on placebo.

Several years later, Pfizer tested their competing drug, Chantix, against Glaxo's Zyban. Pfizer reported that Zyban only helped 16% of smokers quit—this figure is even lower than the results Glaxo gave for the placebo in their tests!

While these drugs are not very effective in helping smokers, they can be counted on to have adverse effects in 100% of people. Bupropion can cause seizures—this effect actually caused it to be unpopular as an antidepressant. This drug frequently causes insomnia, and commonly causes mind-altering effects including abnormal dreams, agitation, anxiety, nervousness, difficulty concentrating, and depression.

The patient and family should be aware of any mental changes as they could mistakenly be diagnosed as new or additional mental illness. Persons already being treated for a mental condition may be at higher risk for the mind-altering effects of this drug.

Other possible mental effects include confusion, hallucinations, delusions, paranoia, restlessness, irritability, hostility, aggression, abnormal dreams, and memory loss. This drug can cause depersonalization where the patient does not feel like her-/himself, and feels “it’s all unreal.”

Bupropion can cause Parkinsonism, with tremors and inability to control muscles. It can cause tardive dyskinesia: a permanent state of drug-induced lack of muscle control with unpredictable jerky movements of the muscles in the face, arms, and legs.

People who are already under treatment with another psychotropic drug may be at greater risk for the mind-altering effects of bupropion. [25]

Chantix (varnicline) attaches to specialized sites on brain cells, partially blocking one of the many locations where nicotine normally acts. It also affects other neurotransmitters. Chantix can cause serious and lasting mental derangement even in people who do not have any prior psychiatric diagnosis. Chantix use is associated with suicidal ideation, suicide attempt, and completed suicide. These mental changes can happen whether or not the patient actually quits smoking, and mental symptoms can continue long after Chantix is stopped.

Chantix may cause depression, homicidal ideation (the urge to murder), mood changes, psychosis, hallucinations, paranoia, delusions, hostility, agitation, anxiety, and panic. Chantix causes changes in behavior, hostility, agitation, irritability, restlessness, depression, and suicidal thinking. The patient and family must be alert to these possible drug effects so as not to mistakenly label them as mental illness. The symptoms may continue even after Chantix is stopped.

Chantix has lately been the number one prescription drug reported to the FDA for being associated with accidents, injury, and death from injury. It is not allowed for people in safety positions, including pilots and missile crews. Users have reported car accidents, near-miss incidents in traffic, and other accidental injuries. In some of these cases, the Chantix user reported excessive sleepiness, dopiness, dizziness, blacking out, or difficulty concentrating. Chantix use has been associated with weakness, amnesia, migraine headache, hyperactivity and restlessness, fainting, tremor, aggression, and difficulty speaking.

The package insert indicates it is necessary to quit smoking for the drug to work. In a study done by Pfizer, the maker of Chantix, 45% of subjects left the study before it was complete. Pfizer reports on the success rate of the remaining people: about 45% stayed off cigarettes for 12 weeks. This gives a false picture of how well the drug actually works. In fact, only 29% of the people who started on Chantix were smoke-free at 12 weeks, and only 16% stayed off cigarettes for an entire year. [26]

The FDA removed the Black Box warnings from the smoking cessation drugs in December 2016. "Black Boxes" are prominent warnings in bold print, outlined with a black border. They are designed to get the attention of doctors so that they will warn their patients of the deadliest possible drug effects. Another purpose of the Black Box is so that doctors will be more watchful for the worst of the drug effects—namely, things that could kill or maim for life.

Black Box warnings about life threatening mental derangement was mandated in 2009 in response to a growing number of spontaneous reports of significant suicidal and violent behaviors, particularly in people on Chantix. In all cases, there was a close relationship to the start of the drug and the change in behavior. Many consumer advocates are outraged at the FDA decision.

"Despite the FDA's error in judgment, patients and physicians need to know that Chantix can cause violent and suicidal behavior, paranoia and psychosis – often beginning soon after starting the treatment, and in people with no previous history of any psychiatric disorder," said Thomas J. Moore, senior scientist with the Public Citizen, the Institute for Safe Medication Practices (ISMP) and a leading expert on Chantix side effects. [27]

The FDA required the drug makers Pfizer and Glaxo to conduct more studies on the mental effects. The company-sponsored study, called EAGLE, incredibly showed no increased incidence of serious mental effects. In September 2016, the FDA convened a panel of "experts," including participants from the drug industry, to review the EAGLE study and the earlier medical reports on the drugs. The panel tore into the studies and found them riddled with inaccuracies and bias. Here is just a sampling of what they found wrong—decide for yourself if you think the study is valid.

Inaccurate and incomplete reporting:

Example 1: A participant had a skull fracture, which was determined to be unrelated to the drug, but it turned out to be inflicted by being hit with a gun by her boyfriend, who was also a study participant. This was not reported as an adverse drug effect for either him or her.

Not counting obvious drug effects:

For example, some study participants reported that depression was so profound that they were missing work or even had to be hospitalized, but such episodes were rated as "mild" by the interviewers.

A 45-year-old study subject took varenicline for 30 days. On day 23, she started hearing voices, became irritable and had trouble thinking, and nightmare and paranoia. Her scores on three rating scales worsened significantly (for anxiety, depression, and general mental state). They had to stop the drug, and then documented that her scores improved significantly. This was not reported as a drug side effect.

Changing the patient's words

There were instances of patients directly reporting dangerous feelings that the FDA was monitoring, such as "anger" and "agitation." Instead, these symptoms were noted by study investigators as vague mood shifts or simply restlessness. This kept them out of the countable category of serious mental effects.

Splitting up the categories:

An adverse drug effect is called "very common" if it occurs in more than 1 in 10 people. A drug effect is termed "frequent" if it occurs in 1 in 10 down to 1 in 100, infrequent if it occurs in more than 1 in 101 to 1 in 1000, and rare if between 1 in 1001 and 1 in 10,000.

In order to stay well out of the "very common" side effect category, the drug companies separate out different kinds of reactions, even though the usual person would lump them together. They separate out neuropsychiatric reactions into separately reportable sections for headache, anxiety, depression, mood changes, and sleep disturbances. That way, each one individually is only reported to happen in 1 to 3% of cases, putting it in the merely "frequent" category. Taken as a whole, the number of neuropsychiatric side effects would add up to "very common," occurring in more than 1 out of every 10 people.

Inconsistent results from center to center:

The largest site reported a 15% rate of serious mental drug effects, but the second largest site, recorded 0 events. In fact, in a sampling of 105 of the centers, there were 60 sites that reported 0 neuropsychiatric events. This was hard for even the FDA to swallow—their own statistical analysis shows this was highly unlikely to happen by chance. Instead, it is a reflection of how much variation there is when it is up to the investigator to decide what constitutes a reaction and its severity.

Financial influence:

The study was funded by Pfizer, maker of Chantix. The study was conducted in several different sites, in multiple countries. The facilities with no financial involvement reliably found more mental drug side effects than the sites that did have financial involvement—up to three and a half times more.

Independent of the monies received by the institutions, many individual study investigators were also in the pay or had been in the pay of Pfizer. At just two sites, for example, there were as many as 60 reports of separate honoraria for speaking engagements and consulting fees. A number of investigators were also receiving ongoing payments from Pfizer for involvement in speaking engagements or other activities not necessarily related to Chantix. This included 39 investigators at 27 sites outside the US and 4 investigators at 4 US sites. [28]

Drugs for Drugs: Psychiatric Drugs to Treat Addiction

The most blatantly irrational use of psychoactive drugs is prescribing narcotics to treat narcotic addiction. The idea is that by giving controlled doses of a narcotic resulting in a lesser high, the patient's craving will be satisfied and they won't go seeking heroin, amphetamines, oxycontin, or morphine.

The model drug has been methadone, a synthetic (man-made) opioid. Synthetics activate the same brain biochemical receptors as plant-based opiates, namely morphine and heroin. Methadone causes less of a high and has a longer duration of action, thus easing the sharp withdrawal symptoms for a heroin addict. However, methadone itself is highly addictive, and it is easy to overdose. There are over 4,000 deaths per year from methadone overdose, despite only being dispensed to registered patients at methadone centers. Methadone can cause all of the typical heroin psychotropic effects, including profound sleepiness, chronic fatigue, weakness, and exhaustion, but also trouble sleeping and insomnia. Methadone causes disorientation, hallucinations, confusion, mood swings, anxiety, panic and fear, memory loss, restlessness, and agitation. [29]

A much bigger problem drug is buprenorphine. Bup, as it is called on the street, is another opioid that is similar to, but somewhat weaker than, morphine or heroin. Bup is a blockbuster drug that outsells big names like Viagra and Adderall. It can cause a high and is easy to become addicted to. Unlike methadone, which is directly given out to registered patients at specially licensed methadone centers, Bup is available by prescription from neighborhood pain doctors' offices. Therefore, there is a high rate of drug diversion (obtaining or creating multiple prescriptions and then selling the drugs). Another factor is that physicians who set themselves up as addiction specialists to be Bup prescribers have a remarkably higher incidence of illegal activity than physicians in other specialties.

It can cause anxiety, depression, dizziness and headaches, nervousness, insomnia, or excessive sleepiness. [30]

When it is stopped, it causes withdrawal symptoms that parallel heroin withdrawal; symptoms can last for months, depending on how long it was abused prior to stopping. [31]

Bup is now being called "prison heroin" because of how it gets smuggled into jails. It can easily be dissolved onto pages of bibles, and the pages eaten; prisoners' blood levels of the drug have shown very adequate absorption to get a high. The Centers for Disease Control (CDC) estimates that some 1,500 children under age 6 were seen in emergency rooms for accidental Bup poisoning in 2010-2011. [32]

For all age groups, emergency department visits involving buprenorphine increased substantially as availability of the drug increased (from 3,161 in 2005 to 30,135 visits in 2010). Over half of those emergencies were from illicit use of the drug not related to a legitimate prescription. [33]

How well does it work? For hard-core addicts, one study showed relapse to heroin occurs in more than 50% of patients within two weeks of tapering off of Bup. [34] A Harvard study showed 78% of young adults relapsed by the three-month mark. [35]

There are no reliable statistics of Bup addiction, mostly because it is accepted medical practice to keep a former heroin addict on Bup for months, years, or indefinitely. Meanwhile, costs of maintaining someone on Bup, for the meds and associated support expenses, ranges from $14,600 to $21,000 per year as of a 2014 report. [36]

In an attempt to reduce the potential for abusing straight Bup, it is combined with naloxone, a drug that blocks the opioid receptors. The combo drug is sold as Suboxone. In prescribed doses, Suboxone allows Bup to attach to opioid receptors, but if the Suboxone is injected or taken in large doses, the naloxone is supposed to block the major effects of Bup. However, it does not work in a textbook fashion and it is still possible to get addicted to the combo preparation. In fact, the incidence of Suboxone addiction is on a sharp rise. [37] The drug distributor, Reckitt Benckiser, promotes Suboxone as a wonder drug to treat heroin addiction, while the reality is that it has become yet another street drug causing addiction. [38]

Virtually no patient under medical addiction treatment is on one psychoactive drug only. Addicts commonly get prescribed benzodiazepines (Xanax and others) to subdue the anxiety and restlessness and to treat the insomnia that typically occurs during withdrawal. However, the benzodiazepines themselves can be addictive after as little as three weeks of continuous use; after long term daily use, benzos can be even more difficult to come off of than the original drug of abuse (such as cocaine or heroin). Alcohol dependence in particular is very commonly treated with benzodiazepines.

Doctors readily assign psychiatric labels to recovering addicts such as anxiety disorder, sleep disorder, depression, thought disorder; all justifying the prescribing of a host of psychiatric drugs. [39] Many people successfully recovered from alcoholism or from the use of illicit drugs are forever after under the effect of regularly prescribed psychoactive drugs. [40]

There are three serious problems with using psychiatric drugs to treat addiction:

1. Relapse rates show they don't work very well for addiction in the first place.
2. Psychiatric replacement drugs can bring on intentional overdose, as they all carry prominent warnings about increased risks of suicide even in people who were not suicidal before taking the drug.
3. When the person reverts to their original drug of abuse, they also have an additional psychoactive drug on board, and the combos can be easier to accidentally overdose on.

Drugs for dementia

Drugs used to treat Alzheimer's are not classified as psychiatric drugs per se, yet they are indeed psychiatric drugs since they are prescribed with the intention to affect mood, emotion, behavior, and thinking. The poster drug in this class is Aricept (donepezil), an inhibitor of the brain neurotransmitter acetylcholine. Related drugs include Exelon (rivastigmine), Razadine (galantamine), and Reminyl (galantamine). This class of chemical was originally discovered when found to be the active ingredient in poisons and venoms that paralyzed the nerves. The acetylcholine inhibitors were initially used as biological warfare agents, aka nerve gas.

Aricept and related drugs prevent the breakdown of acetylcholine, one of the most common messenger chemicals in the body. This is based on a theory that dementia happens because of a lack of acetylcholine. In fact, the package insert for Aricept, the best-selling dementia drug in the world, states:

"There is no evidence that donepezil [Aricept®] alters the course of the underlying dementing process."

Aricept and related drugs frequently cause:

- delusions
- tremor
- irritability
- restlessness
- abnormal crying
- nervousness
- aggression
- a feeling that room is spinning
- numbness
- insomnia
- unbalanced walking
- abnormally increased sex drive
- inability to speak

Other symptoms reported while on dementia drugs include:

- hostility
- emotional instability
- emotional withdrawal
- rapid jerking of eyeballs
- pacing
- nerve pain
- depressed mood
- muscle spasm
- inability to walk
- stiff muscles or lax muscles
- paranoia
- difficulty forming words
- difficulty swallowing

Family and caregivers should be aware of these frequent mental and neurological side effects so the symptoms are not mistakenly assigned to just more dementia or new mental illness.

Patients who take Aricept or related drugs for dementia have a similar range of responses as people who take a dummy pill: the majority stay the same, but some get a little worse, some get a little better; a small percentage get moderately worse and a small percentage get moderately better. Very few get significantly worse and very few get significantly better. The measuring tools used by the drug maker to see if patients got any better were largely based on patient interviews that were not standard (not the same from interviewer to interviewer), so the results cannot be called scientific. [41]

Ebixa and Namenda are composed of memantine, a drug that antagonizes the neurotransmitter NMDA. NMDA antagonists are in the same general drug class as the hallucinogens, including PCP (angel dust) and ketamine. These drugs affect many different brain areas and several additional brain messenger chemicals besides NMDA.

How the drug is supposed to work is not known. In fact, the manufacturer admits there is no evidence these drugs prevent or slow brain degeneration in Alzheimer's.

The NMDA antagonist drugs carry a prominent warning about severe psychiatric symptoms.

Namenda or Ebixa use has been associated with confusion, hallucination, insomnia, depression, anxiety, excessive sleepiness or agitation, self-injury, and aggression.

Namenda and Ebixa may also cause: [42]

- terrifying dreams
- delusions
- personality changes
- paranoia
- suicide attempt
- apathy
- changes in appetite
- abnormal crying
- unstable mood
- increased sexual interest
- numbness
- convulsions
- abnormal body movements
- involuntary muscle contractions
- abnormal coordination
- nerve damage
- drooping eyelids
- numbness
- tingling
- weakness
- bleeding into the brain
- stroke

The family and caregivers must be alert to these drug effects so they are not mistakenly blamed on worsening Alzheimer's.

Namenda drug studies submitted to the FDA for its approval in the US included a total of 418 Alzheimer subjects taking the drug, with studies going for 12 to 28 weeks.

1. The long-term safety of this drug is not known.
2. It acts in the brain like PCP.
3. Jacking up our elderly on hallucinogens was worth some $1.6 billion dollars in annual Namenda sales before going generic in 2015.

It is wise to remember: any drug that causes a change in mind, mood, emotion, or behavior is, by definition, a psychotropic agent, regardless of whether it is prescribed in a psychiatric setting.

CHAPTER 13

Mental Effects of Some Common Medical Drugs

In this era of 5-minute clinic visits and big-box pharmacies, it is more important than ever for patients to get themselves informed of possible drug effects. All too often the affected patient and their prescribing physician are not aware of the potential for sometimes severe derangements in mood, emotion, thought processes, and behaviors that can be caused by usual (non-psychiatric) medical drugs. This can easily result in misidentification of symptoms as a primary psychiatric problem, leading to psychiatric drugging, when the only thing needed is for the offending drug to be stopped. In the worst-case scenario, a mental change caused by a medical drug can deliver a previously sane person into lifelong psychiatric treatment.

Consider the case of Allan Woolley, a 53-year old schoolmaster from Hampstead, England who had no psychiatric history. He was prescribed the cholesterol-lowering drug Zocor (simvastatin), which gave him nightmares, hallucinations, and blackouts. He was killed when he positioned himself on the train tracks at a commuter station, holding a note that read: "Just burn my wretched body without ceremony."

His family maintained this was entirely out of character for him, and an inquest was held. The jury concluded: "At the time of his death Allan Woolley was suffering from psychic disturbances, a known side-effect of the drug simvastatin." [1]

Drugs for Heart and Blood Pressure

Statin drugs such as Crestor (rosuvastatin), Zocor (simvastatin), Pravachol (pravastatin), and Lipitor (atorvastatin) penetrate into the brain to varying degrees, depending on their molecular configuration. In the short run, the anti-inflammatory effect of statins seems to protect against dementia. But after a few years, there is some evidence that statin drugs may actually increase dementia. This may be because cholesterol is a fundamental component of the walls and lining of nerve and brain cells. Stripping the brain of its cholesterol could slow down nerve impulses. All of the statin drugs have the potential to cause mental effects, including memory loss, forgetfulness, amnesia, and confusion. Personality changes with severe mental instability have been reported.

Patients should be aware of these possible side effects so they are not mistakenly labeled with mental illness or Alzheimer's.[2]

The potential for statins to affect dementia are discussed at length in the eBook *A No-nonsense Guide to Cholesterol Medications.* [3]

Drugs for blood pressure and heart disease often act at central locations in the brain, as well as acting locally on the vessels and heart fibers. The blood pressure lowering medications Norvasc (amlodipine), Procardia (nifedipine), and related drugs block the flow of calcium across cell membranes, thereby interrupting numerous basic reactions in the body. These calcium channel blockers can sometimes cause low mood such as apathy or depression, fatigue and sleepiness, or can cause nervousness and insomnia. Norvasc, Procardia, and related drugs can cause male or female sexual dysfunction, abnormal dreams, anxiety, and depersonalization (where a patient does not recognize that he is causing his own actions). Calcium channel blocking drugs can affect the memory, all the way to causing full amnesia. These drugs can cause muscle twitching, unsteady movements, and inability to coordinate. [4]

Another class of drugs lowers the blood pressure by affecting an enzyme found throughout the body, including in the kidneys, brain, and on blood vessels. The so-called ACE inhibitors, such as Capoten (captopril), Vasotec (enalapril), Accupril (quinapril), Lotensin (benazepril), Prinivil and Zestril (lisinopril), and others can all cause mental effects, including memory impairment, confusion, insomnia, sleepiness and sleeping excessively, irritability, and nervousness. [5]

Catapres (clonidine) and Cardura (doxazosin) act directly in the brain to stimulate the lowering of blood pressure. Clonidine's profound mental side effects have led to its use as a primary psychiatric drug. Mood altering drugs similar to Catapres are covered in chapter 8. Cardura can cause fatigue, sleepiness, anxiety, insomnia, nervousness, depression, sexual dysfunction, confusion, and muscle twitching. [6]

Corgard (nadolol) and related drugs block the so-called beta receptors found at various locations including heart and blood vessels. Corgard and related beta-blocker drugs can cause depression progressing all the way to a state of catatonia (immobile and not responsive, yet awake). Beta-blockers can cause hallucinations, disorientation for time and place, short-term memory loss, and emotional instability with unclear thinking. [7]

Blood pressure drugs that block the receptors for a transmitter called angiotensin act on the blood vessels directly, but also at receptor sites in the kidneys and brain. Angiotensin receptor blockers such as Cozaar (losartan), Benicar (olmesartan), and Atacand (candesartan) can cause mental effects including anxiety, nervousness, panic, confusion, depression, weird and vivid dreams, decreased sexual interest, memory impairment, sleep problems, excessive sleepiness, tremor, and dizziness. [8]

Drugs for Gastrointestinal Disorders

Receptors for most neurotransmitters can be found in the digestive tract, as well as in the brain. The stomach, small bowel, and colon each have their own neural network with specialized nerve cells. They sense stretch and tension, mechanical bulk, pressure, temperature, water concentration, and chemical irritation. Motor nerves located in the gut control the movement of food throughout the processes of digestion and elimination, and control constriction, absorption of water, and secretion of gut hormones and digestive enzymes. Norepinephrine, acetylcholine, histamine, and serotonin are some of the neurotransmitters involved in the gut nervous system. It is no surprise, then, that stomach medications commonly cause mental side effects.

Nexium (esomeprazole) and related drugs such as Protonix (pantoprazole) and Prilosec (omeprazole) inhibit the hydrogen-pumping mechanism in the stomach. Any of these drugs can cause aggression, agitation, depression, and hallucinations. [9]

Histamine-blockers like Zantac (ranitidine) and Tagamet (cimetidine) can cause weakness, sleepiness or insomnia, dizziness or vertigo, mental confusion, agitation, involuntary muscle jerking, depression, and hallucinations. [10]

Reglan (metoclopramide) is given for nausea and for slow digestion as is often seen in diabetes. Reglan carries a Black Box warning about tardive dyskinesia, where uncontrollable repetitive muscle jerking, facial grimacing, and tongue contortions can be disabling or even permanent despite stopping the drug. Reglan can cause hallucinations, psychosis, suicidality, agitation, insomnia, and neuroleptic malignant syndrome with high fever and rapid mental deterioration, which can progress to coma and death. [11]

The anti-nausea drugs Zofran (ondansetron) and Kytril (granisetron) block serotonin. They can cause sedation, anxiety, agitation, and movement disorders, especially involving the eyes and face. Serotonin syndrome can occur with symptoms of agitation, hallucinations, delirium and coma, fast heart rate, unstable blood pressure, dizziness, profuse sweating, flushing and high fever, tremors, or muscle stiffness. [12]

The anti-nausea drugs Phenergan (promethazine) and Compazine (prochlorperazine) are phenothiazine drugs that only differ slightly in molecular structure from the first-generation neuroleptic drugs. They can cause hallucinations, psychosis, dyskinesia, Parkinson's-like movement disorders, and neuroleptic malignant syndrome.

Parkinson's Drugs

Parkinson's disease is caused by an actual measured deficiency of dopamine in the brain. All drugs for Parkinson's are directed at increasing available dopamine or enhancing dopamine activity. They manage to accomplish this, but it turns out that just like with the neuroleptic drugs, monkeying with the brain's dopamine can be predicted to also cause mental symptoms. All of the Parkinson's drugs do so, especially with long-term use. Conversely, all psychotropic drugs that affect dopamine can cause Parkinson's-like movement disorders.

The major Parkinson's drugs consist of levodopa in various combinations, such as Sinamet and Stalevo. These drugs carry a major warning about drug-induced depression and suicidality. Sinemet or Stalevo can cause the user to fall asleep suddenly without any prior drowsiness—this can happen during driving, eating, or talking; leading to car accidents, choking, and falls. The mental side effects of dopamine-enhancing drugs are the same as those for the neuroleptic drugs and include dyskinesia (uncontrolled jerking of the extremities and face). Neuroleptic malignant syndrome (NMS) can occur, especially during dosage reductions or when stopping the drug. NMS gives a very high fever, muscle rigidity, and mental derangement that can progress to coma and death.

Sinemet, Stalevo, and related drugs frequently cause excessive and vivid dreams. They cause hallucinations, which may progress to full blown psychosis with confusion and insomnia. These drugs can cause disordered thinking with paranoia, delusions, disorientation, aggressive behavior, agitation, and delirium; impaired memory, anxiety, restlessness, and a sense of euphoria; intense urges to gamble, increased sexual urges, intense urges to spend money or binge eat, and the inability to control these urges. [13]

Azilect (rasagiline) and Eldepryl (selegiline) are Parkinson's drugs that inhibit the enzyme monoamine oxidase. It is not known how this ends up enhancing brain dopamine. The adverse effects are the same as for the levodopa drugs described above.

Requip and Mirapex are also used for Parkinson's disease, and the mental effects of those drugs are discussed in the section on restless legs syndrome in chapter 12.

Drugs to Treat Infections

Drugs to treat infections due to viruses, bacteria, fungus, and parasites all have the potential to cause unwanted mental effects. The antiviral drug Tamiflu (oseltamivir) inhibits an enzyme in viruses. Tamiflu use has been associated with sudden bizarre behaviors like agitation, anxiety, violence, and suicide, especially in children. Patients on Tamiflu have become confused, delirious, and have reported hallucinations and nightmares.

Patients and families should be aware of these possible mental effects so they are not blamed on the flu or mental illness.

It is estimated by the Centers for Disease Control that more than 90% of flu strains were resistant to Tamiflu in 2009. This is because generations of virus particles have mutated to no longer be affected by the enzyme-blocking action of the drug. Even before the resistant strains were discovered, the best Tamiflu ever did was shorten illness by 1 day in the elderly, by 1.3 days in adults, and by 1.5 days in children, and only if it was taken in the first 48 hours of symptoms. [14]

Interferons are another group of anti-viral drugs that are also used to treat hepatitis C, multiple sclerosis, and in some cancer treatments. Interferons can cause depression, with interferon-alpha being more likely to cause this than interferon-beta. Patients on interferon may develop delirium, mania, and psychotic syndromes requiring the treatment to be stopped. [15]

Among antibiotics, the most notorious for causing mental effects are the quinolones, including such drugs as Cipro (ciprofloxacin), Floxin (ofloxacin), and Avelox (moxifloxacin). These drugs can cause nerve damage in the hands, arms, legs, and feet, but they also affect the brain. Due to lack of recognition of drug side effects, it is certain that quinolone-induced mental effects are vastly underreported. These drugs can cause extreme tiredness and intense fatigue, brain fog, depression, short-term memory loss, and depersonalization (a feeling that all is unreal, one is not oneself). The quinolones can cause slurred speech, inability to speak fluently, forgetting of words, and getting stuck in the middle of a sentence. [16]

The investigative journalist Stephen Fried wrote an entire book about the mental experiences of his wife after taking just one tablet of Floxin. She became delirious, disoriented, and unable to function. The symptoms settled into a harrowing three-year experience of an emotional roller coaster resembling manic-depression. [17]

Anti-malarial drugs such as Lariam (mefloquine) are used to prevent and treat malaria as well as other parasite infections. Lariam is routinely given to military personnel serving in Somalia, Iraq, and Afghanistan. It is also used for travelers visiting areas where malaria is found based on recommendations from the Centers for Disease Control and Prevention. The FDA has recently required stronger warning language on the package insert for these drugs. Lariam and related drugs can cause psychiatric and neurological effects that can last for months to years after the drug is stopped, or they can be permanent. They may cause dizziness, balance problems, and ringing in the ears, convulsions or seizures, insomnia, anxiety, paranoia, hallucinations, depression, restlessness, confusion, and personality changes. [18]

Miscellaneous Drugs with Mental Effects

Antihistamines act by blocking the action of the neurotransmitter histamine. There are four main types of histamine receptors found in various tissues throughout the body, including several areas in the brain; on white blood cells; in the nose, throat, and mouth; on smooth muscles; on the lining of the stomach and gut; and on blood vessels. Histamines are most well known as being major players in immune responses such as causing a runny nose with allergies, but they also act in the brain by helping to regulate sleep and wakefulness. Histamine is so widely distributed in the brain that it is presumed to have other important functions yet to be determined. Benadryl (diphenhydramine) is an example of a first generation antihistamine that can cause profound sleepiness. The first generation antihistamine drugs have recently been demonstrated to promote the early onset of dementia when used daily for as little as three years. [19]

The second generation antihistamines don't have this effect. Claritin (loratidine) instead can cause insomnia, restlessness, and nervousness. [20]

The cough suppressant dextromethorphan is found in Robitussin, Vicks-44, and hundreds of other cold remedies. It is usually well tolerated at recommended dosages, but can cause severe mental effects when it is abused or used with other drugs.

Dextromethorphan can cause:[21]

extreme sensitivity to sensations in the environment	a weird sense of disassociation from one's body
visual hallucinations	impaired judgment and mental performance
loss of coordination	extreme tiredness or hyperactivity
slurred speech	euphoria (high feeling)
panic attacks	extreme paranoia
seizures	

Steroids are well known for sometimes causing extreme anger responses uncharacteristic for the patient; this is especially likely when very high doses are used such as by body builders. So-called "roid rage" can progress to homicide and suicide. The doctor of world heavyweight wrestling champion Chris Benoit was providing him with excessive prescriptions for anabolic (muscle-building) steroids in very high doses along with Xanax and hydrocodone. Benoit suffocated his young son, strangled his wife, and hung himself from his exercise equipment. While he may have had some component of traumatic brain injury from concussions over the years, the autopsy of his brain showed over twenty times the normal amount of testosterone—no doubt from the steroids. This alone is enough to make anyone a homicidal-suicidal maniac. [22] But even when steroids are used in usual dosages for medical conditions, they can cause severe mood instability ranging from euphoria to severe depression, or can cause insomnia, personality changes, psychotic manifestations with personality changes, and hallucinations. [23]

Isotretinoin was formerly sold as Accutane and is still available under various brand names. It is a prescription acne medication that bears a close resemblance to retinoic acid: a naturally occurring form of vitamin A present in small amounts in the body. Animal models show isotretinoin disrupts brain nerve transmissions and interferes with serotonin machinery. It can cause psychiatric symptoms including aggressive and violent behaviors, psychosis and depression leading to suicidal ideation, suicide attempts, and completed suicides. In a study of over 5,000 patients on isotretinoin, it was found that suicide attempts were more than one and a half to nearly twice as frequent as what would be expected in the population. The increased risk of suicidality extended for at least six months after stopping the drug, which is how long the patients were followed. It remains unknown how long the mental effects really last. [24]

In a unique and very effective model of risk management, the US FDA requires any dermatologist wishing to write a prescription for isotretinoin must register their patient on a website called iPLEDGE. Pharmacists must then verify the prescription on the website before dispensing. However, the website focuses on informing about birth defects rather than the psychiatric drug effects. [25]

This has been just a partial listing of some common non-psychiatric medical drugs that frequently cause mental effects. It is important to routinely demand full informed consent from your doctor or pharmacist, and then do your own research into potential adverse drug effects.

CHAPTER 14

CONSUMER BEWARE

How can the average health care consumer be protected from adverse drug effects? First and foremost, it is necessary to abandon the notion that every sign of distress needs to be answered with a prescription. It is a simple matter of not putting yourself in harm's way unnecessarily, which you do every time you pop a pill.

Be willing to look at lifestyle habits and your environment to identify accumulated stressors that predisposed you to mental anguish or precipitated a crisis, such as alcohol and drugs, poor eating habits, lack of exercise, extended schedules of long duration, negative persons in the vicinity. You may find you've been living a life that has nothing to do with your true purposes. A doctor's office is the least likely place someone in spiritual distress is going to get listened to and helped. Family and/or clergy are traditional sources of emotional succor and will serve you better than any doctor's office.

Secondly, remember that your doctor works for you. You may have no choice but to pay for government-mandated insurance and fork over the deductible and co-pays, but don't relinquish responsibility for decisions around accepting questionable diagnoses and treatments. Cultivate the intention, and habit, of extracting just what you need from the doctor's education and experience. Above all, be alert that your expertise exceeds that of the doctor when it comes to your own mental health—no matter what a doctor may say or imply to the contrary. The prevailing healthcare model is strictly pharmaceutical and surgical; any complaint will be "medicalized" and addressed as just so much biochemistry and anatomy. Lifestyle changes, powerful nutritional handlings, and a thoughtful examination of stressors in the home and work environments are not anything doctors are trained in, much less have the time or inclination to share with you. The typical five-to-seven minute doctor visit is entirely inadequate to thoroughly listen to a patient's upsetting issues or to provide counsel on non-drug alternatives.

When confronted with a person with mental symptoms, most doctors will not even attempt to do what they are trained in—namely, sort out if there is an underlying medical condition causing or aggravating emotional upset.

The list of medical conditions that can give mental effects is very long, but the most common are the following:

vitamin or mineral deficiencies (especially B vitamins, magnesium, vitamin D)	toxicities (such as mercury or lead)
thyroid problems (low or high)	anemia
gluten intolerance	cancer
any variety of food sensitivities	sleep apnea
chronic infections (such as candida, AIDS, Lyme disease)	hormone problems (including diabetes, adrenal fatigue, menopause, menstrual cycle irregularities, testosterone deficiency)

In the very young or the elderly, even a simple illness with a stomach bug or a urinary tract infection can manifest as emotional upset, confusion, or misbehavior.

Finally, prescription drugs are a very common cause of mental symptoms, particularly when there is more than one drug on board. The tendency to skip a thorough physical evaluation in people presenting with emotional upset has been documented to be exceedingly common.

- Over 30% of the time, non-psychiatric physicians who refer a patient for mental treatment miss an easily detectable underlying physical illness.

- Over 50% of physical illnesses are missed by psychiatrists. [1]

Healthcare providers all-too-readily resort to prescribing psychiatric drugs. Sadly, a major reason is that doctors fully expect they cannot really offer anything truly helpful for mental distress. They default to doing the most expedient thing to "move the patient along" by handing out a prescription.

An appropriate use of a doctor is to demand a full physical and basic lab tests, including a chemistry panel, blood count, thyroid tests, vitamin D and B12 levels, and anything else, such as salivary cortisol measurements. It may also be prudent to seek an alternative practitioner for nutritional and other advice, which is beyond the scope of training of a conventional medical doctor.

There are some additional, less obvious but more menacing situations that might be making you a victim of your doctor's overprescribing habits. The usual doctor who is working in a practice of over 2,500 patients with 30 patient visits in a day has little time or inclination to undertake a critical reading of his or her medical journals afterhours. So it is common practice to rely heavily on glossy promotional materials compiled by the drug company. Periodically, there is a new cluster of studies demonstrating that such advertising matter is misleading at best and criminally deceptive at worst. Yet pharmaceutical company advertising continues to be the primary, often only, medical "education" for too many physicians. This is heavily encouraged by the distribution of free sample medications, facilitating a real no-brainer for the clinic to give out a sample and follow up with a prescription. [2]

A diligent reading of select medical journals may not be much better, however. Most medical journals have some sort of conflict of interest policy that applies to authors, but the majority of such policies do not extend to disclosure of conflicts of interest for their reviewers, editors, or publishers. Even many of the non-profit physician organizations that publish journals often receive more revenue from advertising purchased in their journals than from membership fees. The fact is that journals would not be able to survive without advertising. Medical journals whose editors too critically review studies sponsored by the drug industry can experience a substantial loss of advertising revenue. These problems led Richard Smith, editor with the British Medical Journal for 25 years, to conclude that medical journals are "an extension of the marketing arm of pharmaceutical companies." [3]

It is wise to never underestimate the potential reach and influence of conflicts of interest, obvious or not.

Now that you have read about each class of drugs, it would be helpful to return to the introduction and reread the principles of Informed Consent. Always demand full Informed Consent from your doctor—he or she should describe exactly what the drug is and precisely what the drug does. When you find out that the mechanism of action is unknown or only guessed at, ask your doctor why they believe the drug is right for you. You should be told what is known and not known about the drug's effectiveness, or lack thereof, including whether it is being prescribed experimentally, or off-label. The prescribing physician should fully inform you of what is known and not known about potential adverse effects, not the least of which are the FDA-mandated Black Box Warnings and other Special Precautions on the package insert.

A discussion of viable alternatives to the drug is a crucial component of Informed Consent, including information about exercise being as effective as drugs for most cases of depression, for example.

Finally, it is completely reasonable for you to ask for full disclosure of potential conflicts of interest. Typical conflicts of interest could include the clinic staff getting free lunches from the friendly drug sales reps, the doctor holding stock in pharmaceutical companies, or the medical center being paid to enroll patients in a drug study. Many medical offices are stocked with free samples, which encourages them to thoughtlessly give out the drug most readily at hand and follow it up with a very pricey prescription. If the doctor is writing with a pen emblazoned with a drug name, drinking from a coffee mug with a drug company logo, and writing on a pad with a drug logo, you know you are in a heavily influenced office.

Unfortunately, the Internet is even more saturated with drug company interest. By actual survey, a product is being pushed directly or indirectly on 95% of consumer health sites. Sometimes it is evident by rolling your cursor over highlighted key words, which will cause ads to pop up. Other times, you have to probe three clicks deep to see the pharma connection.

Above all, remember that you are still the paying consumer, even though there is a Federal mandate to be insured (such as Obamacare). You have a right to expect the doctor to work for you and that most definitely includes them answering your questions. If he or she does not have time or is offended, find another doctor pronto. In no circumstances should you give up your right to an opportunity for full Informed Consent.

Thank you for reading! Please write a review so others who may benefit from this or any other book in the No-Nonsense Guide series can read your comments.

Please avail yourself of other books in the series:

No-Nonsense Guide to Cholesterol Medications, Informed Consent and Statin Drugs

No-Nonsense Guide to Antibiotics, Dangers, Benefits & Proper Use

NOTES ON DISCONTINUATION OF DRUGS

If discovering the information about various psychiatric drugs has given you second thoughts about taking the medication you are prescribed, it is crucial to heed warnings about a slow taper to get off the drugs. Abruptly stopping can cause severe and even life-threatening withdrawal symptoms. Stopping suddenly can also cause you to go psychotic, as the altered chemical receptors on brain cells have grown dependent on the changes caused by the drug.

The very doctor who is writing your prescriptions is the one who should be responsible for medically managing your taper off in a safe manner. But the horrible truth is that doctors are given free rein to prescribe, but know almost nothing about safe withdrawal. For example, it's unlikely that your prescribing doctor today could rattle off the five most common adverse effects of your drug, or is aware of the main signs of serotonin syndrome. It is doubtful that he or she knows the severe drug-induced nutritional deficiencies that need to be addressed for a successful withdrawal.

Instead, you are likely to be talked into a prescription for an alternate psychiatric drug. Benzodiazepines are the most commonly prescribed drugs for withdrawal symptoms, which are more quickly addictive and cause more wretched withdrawal symptoms than even heroin. If you are tempted to accept this chemical crutch, re-read the Benzodiazepines section of this book in Chapter 7!

See if you can find a doctor (it need not be a psychiatrist) who will work with you to taper off. This may be a so-called "orthomolecular" psychiatrist—one who works mostly with nutritional support rather than drugs. It may be necessary to switch to liquid forms of your drug in order to make the dosage reduction in the appropriately small increments.

There are a few key resources for psychiatric drug withdrawal.

The Road Back website provides a free program with a very detailed and totally free guidebook. This resource describes itself as the most widely used outpatient drug withdrawal program in the world, having helped over 50,000 people to become drug free since 1999. The program includes detailed information on the kinds of things to expect during withdrawal from each class of drug. It includes dosing reduction guidelines and the precise nutritional support that will be needed. The Road Back is a member of the California Association of Alcoholism & Drug Abuse Counselors (CAADAC).

See http://www.theroadback.org/ and their video at https://www.youtube.com/watch?v=j4cKUWgIxUQ

Harm Reduction Guide to Coming Off Psych Drugs is a 40-page guide written by Will Hall with a 14-member health professional advisory board and 24 other collaborators. It is available for free download at the Icarus Project and Freedom Center website:

http://www.freedom-center.org/freedom-center-icarus-project-publish-coming-psychiatric-drugs-guide/ and video at https://www.youtube.com/watch?v=O4bdG601k4k/

Articles on the topic include "Withdrawing Safely from Psychiatric Drugs" by Dr Maureen B. Roberts, who is the Director of the Schizophrenia Drug-free Crisis Centre in South Australia.

See http://www.jungcircle.com/schiznatural.htm/

It includes the broad steps of dosage reduction and the appropriate nutritional supplements to ease the way. She does mention large doses of folic acid, and I would only suggest using the natural methylated form of folate instead of the synthetic.

"Quitting Psychiatric Drugs" is described in a 1-pager found on the Second Opinion Society website at http://www.walnet.org/llf/drugs/psychdrugs1.html#quitting/

Additional videos on withdrawal include Norman Doidge, MD who describes how to accelerate the withdrawal process: https://www.youtube.com/watch?v=jEeNcZ5jzEY/

Dr. Kelly Brogan describes safe drug withdrawal at: https://www.youtube.com/watch?v=R3TEYOzCogM/

Finally, a variety of peer recovery groups may really help. Here are some places to start:

Everything Matters/Beyond Meds: https://beyondmeds.com/2012/12/04/psychiatric-drug-withdrawal/

Mind Freedom: http://www.mindfreedom.org/who-we-are/

Psychiatric Medication Awareness Group: http://www.psychmedaware.org/groups.html

I hope this is helpful. I sincerely wish you a happy and productive future.

ABOUT THE AUTHOR

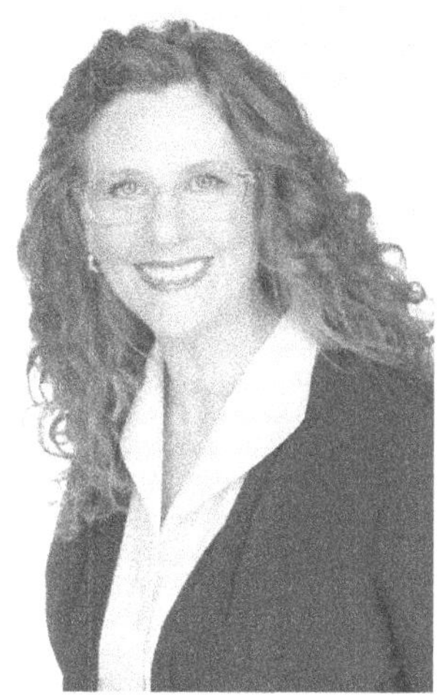

Moira Dolan, MD is a patient-centered physician and champion of Informed Consent, a graduate of the University of Illinois School of Medicine, and certified by the American Board of Internal Medicine as well as by the American Academy of Anti-Aging Medicine. For many years, Dr. Dolan consulted for the Office of the Inspector General in Texas to identify improper treatments and inappropriate medical billing claims, and currently serves as Medical Director of a healthcare audit firm. She has no financial conflicts of interest for forwarding or censuring any particular drug treatment and intentionally sought out service providers for the packaging of this material who also did not have conflicts of interest. Dr. Dolan is director of The Medical Accountability Network and maintains a medical news blog on SmartMEDInfo.com. She lives in Austin, Texas.

ACKNOWLEDGEMENTS

This book is the result of years of work with hundreds of patients and their families who were never given the opportunity for informed consent on psychiatric treatment. When they worsened, they had no inkling that they were suffering from known adverse drug effects ranging from insomnia and depression to violent rage and suicide. All too often the symptoms were attributed to "just more mental illness" and the preventable nature of their downward spiral did not become known until after a tragic event. Their traumas repeatedly demonstrated the need for a plain English reference guide for anyone on or considering taking a psychoactive drug. If this guide can help one person, then perhaps the suffering of many yet yielded some good.

REFERENCES

Chapter 1

1. Lectlaw Library website: http://www.lectlaw.com/def/i038.htm

2. Jones, W H S, translator of Hippocrates' *Ancient Medicine. Airs, Waters, Places. Epidemics 1 and 3. The Oath. Precepts. Nutriment.* Loeb Classical Libraries, 1923.

3. *The Nazi Doctors and the Nuremberg Code: Human Rights in Human Experimentation* Paperback by George J Annas (Editor), Michael A Grodin (Editor). Oxford University Press, August 24, 1995.

4. *World Medical Association Declaration of Helsinki: Ethical Principles for Medical Research Involving Human Subjects.* Adopted by the 18th WMA General Assembly, Helsinki, Finland, June 1964. Available on the World Medical Association website at http://www.wma.net/en/30publications/10policies/index.html

5. "Belmont Report: Ethical Principles and Guidelines for the Protection of Human Subjects of Research" by The National Commission for the Protection of Human Subjects of Biomedical and Behavioral Research is available at the HHSC website at http://www.hhs.gov/ohrp/humansubjects/guidance/belmont.html

Chapter 2

1. Bancroft, J, and I Marks. "Electric aversion therapy of sexual deviations". *Proc R Soc Med.* (Aug 1968) 61(8):796–799.

2. Society of Biological Psychiatry website http://www.sobp.org/i4a/pages/index.cfm?pageid=1

3. Ott, Jonathan. *Pharmacotheon: Entheogenic Drugs, Their Plant Sources.* Natural Products Co 2nd Edition, 1993.

4. Lundie, H. *The Phrenological Mirror; or, Delineation Book.* Leeds: C. Croshaw, 1844.

5. Wagner-Jauregg, J. "Nobel Lecture: The Treatment of Dementia Paralytica by Malaria Inoculation". *Nobel Lectures, Physiology or Medicine 1922-1941.* Elsevier Publishing Company, Amsterdam, 1965.

Chapter 3

1. https://en.wikipedia.org/wiki/Hysteria

2. Tasca, Cecilia, Mariangela Rapetti, Mauro Giovanni Carta, and Bianca Fadda. "Women and Hysteria in the History of Mental Health." *Clin Pract Epidemiol Ment Health* (2012) 8:110–119.

3. http://kheper.net/topics/typology/four_humours.html

4. Hippocrates. *The Nature of Man.* trans. W.H.S. Jones. Loeb Classical Library, London, 1931. v.IV. pp.11-13.

5. Burton, Robert. *The Anatomy of Melancholy, What it is: With all the Kinds, Causes, Symptomes, Prognostickes, and Several Cures of it. In Three Maine Partitions with their several Sections, Members, and Subsections. Philosophically, Medicinally, Historically, Opened and Cut Up.* First published in 1621. T C Faulkner, N K

Kiessling, and R L Blair, eds. Oxford, Clarendon Press. Three Volumes. 1989-1994.

6. Jansson, A. "Mood Disorders and the Brain: Depression, Melancholia, and the Historiography of Psychiatry". *Med Hist* (Jul 2011) 55(3):393–399.

7. Kraeplin, E. *Compendium der Psychiatrie*. Abel Leipzig, 1883. Available in the World Catalogue Database.

8. Deichmann, U. *Biologists Under Hitler*. Harvard University Press, 1999.

9. Healy, D, M Harris, F Farquhar, S Tschinke, and J Noury. "Historical overview: Kraepelin's impact on psychiatry". *Eur Arch Psychiatry Clin Neurosci* (2008) 258 Suppl 2:18–24.

10. *Statistical Manual for the Use of Institutions for the Insane Published in New York in 1918*. Available on Open Library.org at https://openlibrary.org/books/OL6623438M/Statistical_manual_for_the_use_of_institutions_for_the_insane

11. "Nomenclature of Psychiatric Disorders and Reactions". Office of the Surgeon General, Army Service Forces. War Department Technical Bulletin, *Medical 203.* Originally published in *JCLP* (1946) 2:289–296. Republished in *J Clin Psychol* (2000) 56:925–934.

12. American Psychiatric Association. *Diagnostic and Statistical Manual of Mental Disorders* (*DSM-1*). American Psychiatric Press, 1952.

13. American Psychiatric Association. *Diagnostic and Statistical Manual of Mental Disorders* (*DSM-II*). American Psychiatric Press, 1968.

14. American Psychiatric Association. *Diagnostic and Statistical Manual of Mental Disorders* (*DSM-III*). American Psychiatric Press, 1980.

15. American Psychiatric Association. *Diagnostic and Statistical Manual of Mental Disorders* (*DSM-III-R*). American Psychiatric Association, 1987.

16. Hagen, M. *Whores of the Court: The Fraud of Psychiatric Testimony and the Rape of American Justice*. Regan Press, 1997.

17. American Psychiatric Association. *Diagnostic and Statistical Manual of Mental Disorders* (*DSM-IV*). American Psychiatric Press, 1994.

18. American Psychiatric Association. *Diagnostic and Statistical Manual of Mental Disorders* (*DSM-IV-TR*). American Psychiatric Press, 2000.

19. American Psychiatric Association. *Diagnostic and Statistical Manual of Mental Disorders* (*DSM-V*). American Psychiatric Press, 2013.

20. McHugh MD, P, and P Slavney MD. "Mental Illness — Comprehensive Evaluation or Checklist?" *N Engl J Med* (May 17, 2012) 366:1853-1855.

21. Insel, T. "Transforming Diagnosis". December 4, 2014, in his blog on the NIMH website at http://www.nimh.nih.gov/about/director/2013/transforming-diagnosis.shtml

22. "New psychiatric manual, DSM-5, faces criticism for turning 'normal' human problems into mental illness". *The Associated Press* (Wednesday, May 15, 2013).

23. Cosgrove L, and S Krimsky. "A Comparison of DSM-IV and DSM-5 Panel Members' Financial Associations with Industry: A Pernicious Problem Persists". *PLoS Med* 9(3).

Chapter 4

1. Allexander, Franz G, and Sheldon T Selesnick. *The History*

of Psychiatry: An Evaluation of Psychiatric Thought and Practice from Prehistoric Times to the Present. Harper and Row, 1966.

2. Shapiro, Arthur K, and Elaine Shapiro. *The Powerful Placebo: From Ancient Priest to Modern Physician.* Johns Hopkins University Press, Sep 15, 2000.

3. Rush, Benjamin. *Medical Inquiries and Observations, Upon the Diseases of the Mind.* Published by Samuel Merritt in 1785 or 6.

4. Galt, John M. *Essays on Asylums for Persons of Unsound Mind: Second Series.* Printed by Ritchies & Dunnavant, 1853.

5. Savage MD, George, Physician Superintendent to Bethlem Hospital. "On the Treatment of Insanity, More Especially by Drugs" (1878).

6. Anderson, I. "Nightmare on Chelmsford, Sydney." *New Scientist* No.1750 (5 January 1991).

7. Shorter, E, and D Healy. *Shock Therapy: A History of Electroconvulsive Treatment in Mental Illness.* Rutgers University Press, 2013.

8. von Mach, M A, S Meyer, B Omogbehin, P H Kann, and L S Weilemann. "Epidemiological assessment of 160 cases of insulin overdose recorded in a regional poisons unit". *Int J Clin Pharmacol Ther* (2004) 42(5):277–280.

9. Valenstein, E S. *Great and Desperate Cures: The Rise and Decline of Psychosurgery and Other Radical Treatments for Mental Illness.* Basic Books, 1986.

10. Passione, R. *Non solo l'elettroshock: Ugo Cerletti e il rinnovamento della Psichiatria italiana* [Not only electroshock: Ugo Cerletti and renewal of the Italian Psychiatry]. Marco Piccolino (ed). Neuroscienze Controverse: Da Aristotele alla moderna scienza del linguaggio (Torino: Bollati Boringhieri, 2008), 258.

11. Endler, N S. "The Origins of Electroconvulsive Therapy (ECT)". *Convulsive Therapy* 4(1):5 – 23 (1988).

12. Quirke, V. *Collaboration in the Pharmaceutical Industry: Changing Relationships in Britain and France, 1935-1965 (Routledge Studies in the History of Science, Technology and Medicine)*. Edition 1. Taylor & Francis LTD, 2006.

Chapter 5

1. Barrett, Kim E, Susan M Barman, Scott Boitano, and Heddwen Brooks. *Ganong's Review of Medical Physiology, 24th Edition*. McGraw-Hill Professional, Apr 5, 2012.

2. Pert, Candace B, *Molecules Of Emotion: The Science Behind Mind-Body Medicine*. Touchstone, 1992.

3. Package insert for Delysid, Sandoz, Ltd. (1964).

4. Glennon, R, M Dukat, and R Westkaemper. "Serotonin Receptor Subtypes and Ligands". Posted in 2000 in the online journal Neuropsychopharmacology on the website of the American College of Neuropsychopharmacology at https://www.acnp.org/g4/GN401000039/Ch039.html

5. Heninger G, P Delgado, and D Charney. "The revised monoamine theory of depression: A modulatory role for monoamines, based on new findings from monoamine depletion experiments in humans". *Pharmacopsychiatry* (1996) 29:2–11.

6. Mendels J, J Stinnett, D Burns, and A Frazer. "Amine precursors and depression". *Arch Gen Psychiatry* (1975) 32:22–30.

7. Roggenbach, J, B Müller-Oerlinghausen, and L Franke. "Suicidality, impulsivity, and aggression-Is there a link to 5HIAA concentration in the cerebrospinal fluid?" *Psychiatry Res* (2002) 113: 193–206.

8. Kirsch PhD, Irving. *The Emperor's New Drugs: Exploding the Antidepressant Myth.* Basic Books, 2010.

9. Miller, M C and HHP editors. "Understanding Depression". *Harvard Health Publications* (2013).

10. Blumenthal, J A, MA Babyak, K A Moore, et al. "Effects of Exercise Training on Older Patients with Major Depression". *Arch Intern Med* (1999) 159(19):2349-2356.

11. Fournier MA, Jay C, DeRubeis, PhD, Robert J, Hollon, PhD, Steven D, et al. "Antidepressant Drug Effects and Depression Severity: A Patient-Level Meta-analysis". *JAMA* (2010) 303(1):47-53.

12. Lacasse, J R, and J Leo. "Serotonin and Depression: A Disconnect between the Advertisements and the Scientific Literature". *PLoS Medicine* (2005) 1211-1216.

Chapter 6

1. Prozac package insert. Eli Lilly Pharmaceuticals, 1987; Celexa package insert. Forest Laboratories, rev 1/2009; Zoloft package insert. Pfizer, Inc, rev 1/2009.

2. Leung, R. "Prescription For Murder? Did Zoloft Make 12-Year-Old Chris Pittman Murder His Grandparents?" 48 Hours, April 13, 2005. Accessible online at http://www.christopherpittman.org/

3. El-Mallakh, R S, Y Gao, and Jeannie Roberts. "Tardive dysphoria: the role of long term antidepressant use in-inducing chronic depression". *Med Hypotheses* (2011 June) 76(6):769-73.

4. ISMP (Institute for Safe Medical Practices) Newsletter, September 24, 2014 — Data from 2013 Quarters 2 & 3 http://www.ismp.org/QuarterWatch/pdfs/2013Q3.pdf

5. By Andrew Thibault May 6, 2016. Mad in America blog at

https://www.madinamerica.com/2016/05/the-fda-is-hiding-reports-linking-psych-drugs-to-homicides/

6. Viibrid prescribing information. Allergan Pharmaceuticals, 2016.

7. Fetzima prescribing information. Allergan Pharmaceuticals, 2016.

8. Trintellix prescribing information. Takeda Pharmaceuticals America, 2016.

9. Sena, S, S Kazimi, and A Wu. "False-Positive Phencyclidine Immunoassay Results Caused by Venlafaxine and O-Desmethylvenlafaxine". *Clinical Chemistry* (April 2002) vol.48 no.4:676-677.

10. "Phencyclidine". Drug Enforcement Administration, Office of Diversion Control, Drug & Chemical Evaluation Section (January 2013). Available on the DEA website at http://www.deadiversion.usdoj.gov/drug_chem_info/pcp.pdf

11. Effexor package insert. Wyeth Pharmaceuticals, rev 6/06.

12. Brown, A. "Antidepressant Used by Yates Questioned". *The Associated Press* (July 9, 2006).

13. Effexor package insert. Wyeth Pharmaceuticals, rev 6/06.

14. Abrams, T, in a letter from the FDA to Robert Essner, Chairman and Chief Executive Officer of Wyeth Pharmaceuticals Inc dated 12/10/2007. Available on the FDA website at http://www.fda.gov/downloads/Drugs/GuidanceComplianceRegulatoryInformation/EnforcementActivitiesbyFDA/WarningLettersandNoticeofViolationLetterstoPharmaceuticalCompanies/ucm054126.pdf

15. Staff writers. "Bomb-threat doctor may be detained". *Seattle Times* (July 28, 2007).

Chapter 7

1. Chweh, A Y, et al. "Hypnotic action of benzodiazepines: A possible mechanism". *Life Sciences* (30 April 1984) volume 34, issue 18, pages 1763–1768.

2. Longo, L P, and B Johnson. "Addiction: Part I. Benzodiazepines—Side Effects, Abuse Risk and Alternatives". *Am Fam Physician* (2000 Apr 1) 61(7):2121-2128.

3. Xanax package insert. Pfizer, September 2014.

4. Lunesta package insert. Sunovion, May 2014.

Chapter 8

1. Moreno C, G Laje, C Blanco, et al. "National trends in the outpatient diagnosis and treatment of bipolar disorder in youth". *Arch Gen Psychiatry* (2007 Sep) 64(9):1032-9.

2. Depakote prescribing information. AbbVie, January 2015.

3. Lamictal prescribing information. GlaxoSmithKline, December 2014.

4. Calabrese J R, C L Bowden, G Sachs, et al. "Lamictal 605 Study Group A placebo-controlled 18-month trial of lamotrigine and lithium maintenance treatment in recently depressed patients with bipolar I disorder". *The Journal of Clinical Psychiatry* (2003) 64(9):1013-1024.

5. Tegretol package insert. Novartis, September 2014; Trileptal package insert. Novartis, July 2014.

6. Neurontin package insert. Pfizer Parke-Davis, September 2014.

7. Topamax package insert. Janssen Pharmaceuticals, 2009.

8. Gabutti, L, M Gugger, and H P Marti. "Impaired kidney function in lithium therapy". *Ther Umsch* (1998 Sep) 55(9):562-4.

9. Markowitz, GS, J Radhakrishnan, N Kambham, et al. "Lithium nephrotoxicity: a progressive combined glomerular and tubulointerstitial nephropathy". *J Am Soc Nephrol* (2000 Aug) 11(8):1439-48.

10. Lithobid prescribing information. Noven Therapeutics, 10/2011.

Chapter 9

1. Shen, W W. "A history of antipsychotic drug development". *Compr Psychiatry* (1999 Nov-Dec) 40(6):407-14.

2. Li, J. "Genome-wide shRNA screen revealed integrated mitogenic signaling between dopamine receptor D2 (DRD2) and epidermal growth factor receptor (EGFR) in glioblastoma". *Oncotarget* 5(4), 882-893.

3. Veijola J, J Y Guo, J S Moilanen, E Ja¨a¨skela¨inen, et al. (2014) "Longitudinal Changes in Total Brain Volume in Schizophrenia: Relation to Symptom Severity, Cognition and Antipsychotic Medication". *PLoS ONE* 9(7): e101689.

4. Risperdal package insert. Janssen, 2007.

5. Howard L, G Kirkwood, and M Leese. "Risk of hip fracture in patients with a history of schizophrenia". *Br J Psychiatry* (2007) 190:129–134.

6. FDA Drug Safety Communication of 05-03-2016. http://www.fda.gov/Drugs/DrugSafety/ucm498662.htm/

7. Vraylar prescribing information. Allergan Pharmaceuticals, 2016. AND Rexulti prescribing information. Otsuka Pharmaceutical Co, 2015.

8. "FDA Issues Complete Response Letter for Digital Medicine New Drug Application". Business Wire, April 26, 2016. http://www.businesswire.com/news/home/20160426006993/en/FDA-Issues-Complete-Response-Letter-Digital-Medicine/

9. Haller, D. American Academy of Addiction Psychiatry (AAAP) 24th Annual Meeting & Symposium: Abstract 16, presented December 7, 2013, as reported in Medscape online by Melville, N, Atypical Antipsychotics New Drugs of Abuse Medscape December 17, 2013. Available at http://www.medscape.com/viewarticle/817961

Chapter 10

1. Levy F, and M R Dadds. "Stimulant side effects: prefrontal/basal ganglia circuit control at dopamine D1/D2 receptors". *Australas Psychiatry* (2014 Apr) 22(2):179-82.

2. Adderall package insert. Shire USA Inc, 2014.

3. "The FDA Is Hiding Reports Linking Psych Drugs to Homicides" By Andrew Thibault May 6, 2016. Mad In America blog. https://www.madinamerica.com/2016/05/the-fda-is-hiding-reports-linking-psych-drugs-to-homicides/

4. Strattera package insert. Eli Lilly, 2014.

Chapter 11

1. Myerson, A, F Ebaugh, et al, "Fatalities Following Electric Convulsive Therapy: A Report of 2 Cases with Autopsy Findings". *Transactions of the American Neurological Association* (June 1942).

2. Myerson, A. "Borderline Cases Treated by Electric Shock". *American Journal of Psychiatry* (November 1943).

3. Kennedy, C, and D Anchel. "Regressive Electric-Shock

in Schizophrenics Refractory to Other Shock Therapies". *Psychiatric Quarterly* (1948) vol. 22.

4. Gordon, Major Hirsch L. "Fifty Shock Therapy Theories". *Military Surgeon* (November 1948) vol. 103, No. 5.

5. Sament, S. Letter to Clinical Psychiatry News. March 1983.

6. Gorman, J. "The Essential Guide to Psychiatric Drugs". St. Martin's Press, 1990.

7. Horgan, J (U.S. writer). *The Undiscovered Mind: How the Human Mind Defies Replication, Medication, and Explanation.* New York: Touchstone, 1999.

8. FDA, ECT 515(i) Executive Summary Draft p.17, #5.

9. O'Leary, D, E Paykel, C Todd, and K Vardulaki. "Suicide in primary affective disorders revisited: a systematic review by treatment era". *J Clin Psychiatr* (2001) 62:10:804-811.

10. Gombos, Z, A Spiller, G A Cottrell, et al. "Mossy fiber sprouting induced by repeated electroconvulsive shock seizures". *Brain Res* (1999 Oct 9) 844(1-2):28-33.

11. Scott, B W, J M Wojtowicz, and W M Burnham. "Neurogenesis in the dentate gyrus of the rat following electroconvulsive shock seizures". *Exp Neurol* (2000 Oct) 165(2):231-6.

12. Chen, F, T M Madsen, G Wegener, and J R Nyengaard. "Repeated electroconvulsive seizures increase the total number of synapses in adult male rat hippocampus". *Eur Neuropsychopharmacol* (2009 May) 19(5):329-38.

13. Babigian, et al "Epidemiological considerations in ECT". *Arch Gen Psych* (1984) 41:216-253.

14. Kroessler and Fogel, "Electroconvulsive Therapy for Major Depression in the Oldest Old". *Am J of Geriatric Psychiatry* (1993) 1:1:30-37.

15. Gilbert, D, Commissioner, Texas Department of Mental Health and Mental Retardation, 1996.

16. Clarke, G (U.S. writer). *Get Happy: The Life of Judy Garland.* Random House, 2000.

17. Quoted by A E Hotchner in Part 4, Chapter 14 of *Papa Hemingway*. Random House, 1966.

18. Donahue, Anne B. "Electroconvulsive Therapy and Memory Loss: A Personal Journey". *Journal of ECT (Official Journal of the Association for Convulsive Therapy)* (July 2000).

19. Burkhard, P R, F J Vingerhoets, A Berney, et al. "Suicide after successful deep brain stimulation for movement disorders". *Neurology* (2005 Aug 9) 65(3):499-500.

20. Hershey, T, F J Revilla, A Wernle, et al. "Stimulation of STN impairs aspects of cognitive control in PD". *Neurology* (2004) 62:1110—4.

21. Hariz, GM, P Blomstedt, and L O Koskinen. "Long-term effect of deep brain stimulation for essential tremor on activities of daily living and health-related quality of life". *Acta Neurol Scand* (2008 Dec) 118(6):387-94.

22. Hobson, DE, A E Lang, W R Martin, et al. "Excessive daytime sleepiness and sudden-onset sleep in Parkinson disease: a survey by the Canadian Movement Disorders Group". *JAMA* (2002) 287:455—63.

23. Heo, J H, K M Lee, S H Paek, et al. "The effects of bilateral subthalamic nucleus deep brain stimulation (STN DBS) on cognition in Parkinson disease". *J Neurol Sci* (2008 Oct 15) 273(1-2):19-24.

24. Czernecki, V, B Pillon, J L Houeto, et al. "Does bilateral stimulation of the subthalamic nucleus aggravate apathy in

Parkinson's disease?" *J Neurol Neurosurg Psychiatry* (2005) 76:775—9.

25. Drapier, D, S Drapier, P Sauleau, et al. "Does subthalamic nucleus stimulation induce apathy in Parkinson's disease?" *J Neurol* (2006 Aug) 253(8):1083-91.

26. Voon, V, P Krack, A E Lang, et al. "Parkinson's disease, DBS and suicide: a role for serotonin?" *Brain* (2009 Jun 24).

27. Appleby, B S, P S Duggan, A Regenberg, and P V Rabins. "Psychiatric and neuropsychiatric adverse events associated with deep brain stimulation: A meta-analysis of ten years' experience". *Mov Disord* (2008 Aug 15) 23(11):1626.

28. Schupbach, M, M Gargiulo, M L Welter, et al. "Neurosurgery in Parkinson disease: a distressed mind in a repaired body?" *Neurology* (2006) 66:1811—6.

Chapter 12

1. Mundy, Alicia. "Dispensing With the Truth: The Victims, The Drug Companies, and the Dramatic Story Behind the Battle over Fen-Phen". St. Martin's Press, 2001.

2. Suprenza package insert. Akrimax Pharmaceuticals, 6/2013.

3. Qysmia package insert. Vivus, 10/2014.

4. Contrave package insert. Takeda, 2014; Vivitrol (naltrexone) package insert. Alkermes, 2013.

5. Belviq package insert. Arena Pharmaceuticals, 2012.

6. Mirapex package insert. Boehringer Ingelheim, 2013.

7. Requip package insert. GlaxoSmithKline, 2014.

8. Sinemet package insert. Merck, 2014.

9. Parlodel package insert. Novartis, January 2012.

10. Neupro package insert. UCB Inc, 2013.

11. Viegas, J, "Killer Whales on Valium: Common Practice?" Discovery News, April 4, 2014.

12. Klonopin package insert. Genentech, 2013.

13. Fluoxetine prescribing information. Eli Lilly, 2/2009.

14. Lotronex package insert. Prometheus Labs, March 2014.

15. Johnson, EM, W A Lanier, R M Merrill, et al. "Unintentional prescription opioid-related overdose deaths: description of decedents by next of kin or best contact, Utah, 2008-2009". *Gen Intern Med* (2013 Apr) 28(4):522-9.

16. Imitrex prescribing information. GlaxoSmithKline, 2012.

17. Cafergot prescribing information. Sandoz, 2012.

18. CDC Vital Signs www.cdc.gov/VitalSigns

19. Hegmann, Kurt T, M S Weiss, K Bowden, et al. "ACOEM Practice Guidelines: Opioids and Safety-Sensitive Work". Journal of Occupational & Environmental *Medicine* (July 2014) volume 56, issue 7, pages e46–e53.

20. Neurontin prescribing information. Pfizer, September 2014.

21. "Substance Abuse and Mental Health Services Administration". National Survey on Drug Use and Health, 2014.

22. "F.D.A. Toughens Warning Labels for Some Opioid Painkillers" by Sabrina Tavernise. Science Times, March 22, 2016.

23. Lyrica package insert. Parke-Davis, 2013.

24. Catapres package insert. Boehringer-Ingelheim, 2012.

25. Zyban prescribing information. GlaxoSmithKline, August 2011.

26. Chantix prescribing information. Pfizer, October 2014.

27. "FDA Wrong to Remove Chantix's Black Box Warning Based on One Flawed Study, Sets Dangerous Precedent for Future Medication Safety". Public Citizen press release of Dec 19, 2016. http://www.citizen.org/pressroom/pressroomredirect.cfm?ID=10102

28. "FDA Briefing Document: Serious Neuropsychiatric Adverse Events with Drugs for Smoking Cessation." Joint Meeting of the Psychopharmacologic Drugs Advisory Committee and Drug Safety and Risk Management Advisory Committee, held September 14, 2016. http://www.fda.gov/downloads/AdvisoryCommittees/CommitteesMeetingMaterials/Drugs/PsychopharmacologicDrugsAdvisoryCommittee/UCM520103.pdf

29. Modesto-Lowe MD, MPH, Vania, Donna Brooks MS, and Nancy Petry PhD. "Methadone Deaths: Risk Factors in Pain and Addicted Populations". *J Gen Intern Med* (2010 Apr) 25(4): 305–309.

30. Suboxone prescribing information. Reckitt Benckiser Pharmaceuticals Inc, April 2014.

31. "Intelligence Bulletin: Buprenorphine: Potential for Abuse". National Drug Intelligence Center (September 2004). Document ID: 2004-L0424-013.

32. "Notes from the Field: Emergency Department Visits and Hospitalizations for Buprenorphine Ingestion by Children — United States, Morbidity and Mortality Weekly Report". CDC 2010–2011 (January 25, 2013) 62(03);56-56.

33. "The DAWN Report: Emergency Department Visits Involving Buprenorphine. Substance Abuse and Mental

Health Services Administration". Center for Behavioral Health Statistics and Quality (January 29, 2013).

34. Woodcock, E A, L H Lundahl, and M K Greenwald. "Predictors of buprenorphine initial outpatient maintenance and dose taper response among non-treatment-seeking heroin dependent volunteers". *Drug Alcohol Depend* (Jan 1, 2015) volume 146, pages 89-96.

35. Zev Schuman-Olivier MD, Z, Roger Weiss MD, Bettina B Hoeppner MD, Jacob Borodovsky MD, and Mark J Albanese MD. "Emerging adult age status predicts poor buprenorphine treatment retention". *Journal of Substance Abuse and Treatment* (September 2014) volume 47, issue 3, pages 202–212.

36. Khemiri, A, E Kharitonova, V Zah, J Ruby, and M Toumi. "Analysis of buprenorphine/naloxone dosing impact on treatment duration, resource use and costs in the treatment of opioid-dependent adults: a retrospective study of US public and private health care claims". *Postgrad Med* (2014 Sep) 126(5):113-20.

37. Canestrelli, C, N Marie, and F Noble. "Rewarding or aversive effects of buprenorphine/naloxone combination (Suboxone) depend on conditioning trial duration". *Int J Neuropsychopharmacol* (2014 Sep) 17(9):1367-73.

38. Sontag, D, "The Double-Edged Drug: Addiction Treatment With a Dark Side". New York Times.com (Nov. 16, 2013).

39. Smith, J K. "Co-occurring substance abuse and mental disorders: A practitioner's guide". Lanham, MD: Jason Aronson/ Rowman and Littlefield, 2007.

40. Longo, L, and B Johnson. "Addiction: Part I. Benzodiazepines—Side Effects, Abuse Risk and Alternatives". *Am Fam Physician* (2000 Apr 1) 61(7):2121-2128.

41. Aricept prescribing information. Eisai, 2013.

42. Namenda prescribing information. Forest Laboratories, October 2013.

Chapter 13

1. Keilthy, Paul, "'Superdrug' Death Link? Inquest blames cholesterol pills for psychic disturbances". *Camden New Journal* (10 January 2008).

2. Crestor prescribing information. Parke-Davis, 2014.

3. Dolan MD, M. *No-Nonsense Guide to Cholesterol Lowering Drugs*. 2015.

4. Norvasc prescribing information. Pfizer, 2014.

5. Prinivil prescribing information. Merck, 2014.

6. Cardura prescribing information. Pfizer, 2014.

7. Corgard prescribing information. Pfizer, 2013.

8. Cozaar package insert. Merck, 2013.

9. Nexium prescribing information. Astra Zeneca, 2014.

10. Zantac prescribing information. Covis, 2013.

11. Reglan prescribing information. Alaven Pharmaceutical LLC, 2010.

12. Zofran prescribing information. GlaxoSmithKline, 2014.

13. Sinemet prescribing information. Merck, 2014.

14. Tamiflu prescribing information. Genentech, 2014.

15. Patten, S B. "Psychiatric side effects of interferon treatment". *Curr Drug Saf* (2006 May) 1(2):143-50.

16. Over 300 references on quinolone toxicity can be found in "Quinolone Antibiotics Toxicity" July 2005 on the antibiotics.

org website at http://www.antibiotics.org/resources/side-effects .pdf

17. Fried, Stephen. *Bitter Pills*. Bantam, 1998.

18. FDA Drug Safety Communication: "FDA approves label changes for antimalarial drug mefloquine hydrochloride due to risk of serious psychiatric and nerve side effects". 7/29/2013 FDA website at http://www.fda.gov/Drugs/DrugSafety/ucm362227.htm

19. Gray, S L, M L Anderson, S Dublin, J T Hanlon, R Hubbard, R Walker, O Yu, P K Crane, and E B Larson. "Cumulative Use of Strong Anticholinergics and Incident Dementia: A Prospective Cohort Study". *JAMA Intern Med* (2015) 175(3):401-407.

20. Simons, F E R, T G Fraser, J D Reggin, and K J Simons. "Comparison of the central nervous system effects produced by six h-1-receptor antagonists". *Clin Exp Allergy 26* (1996) 1092-7.

21. Ahmed G, Saleem MD, and H Naim. "How many deaths before we put cough syrups behind the counter?" *Perspect Public Health* (2014 Nov) 134(6):309.

22. Omalu, B I, R P Fitzsimmons, J Hammers, and J Bailes. "Chronic traumatic encephalopathy in a professional American wrestler". *J Forensic Nurs* (2010 Fall) 6(3):130-6.

23. Prednisone prescribing information. Bienheim Pharmacal, 2014.

24. Sundström, A, L Alfredsson, G Sjölin-Forsberg, B Gerdén, U Bergman, and J Jokinen. "Association of suicide attempts with acne and treatment with isotretinoin: retrospective Swedish cohort study". *BMJ* (2010) 341.

25. IPLEDGE website: https://www.ipledgeprogram.com/Default.aspx

Chapter 14

1. Koranyi, E and W Potocznyb. "Physical Illnesses Underlying Psychiatric Symptoms". *Psychother Psychosom* (1992) 58:155-160.

2. Ruiz, R. "Ten Misleading Drug Ads". Posted 2/02/2010 on Forbes.com.

3. Smith, R. "Medical Journals Are an Extension of the Marketing Arm of Pharmaceutical Companies". *PLoS Med* 2(5):e138.

www.ingramcontent.com/pod-product-compliance
Lightning Source LLC
Chambersburg PA
CBHW060337030426
42336CB00011B/1379

* 9 7 8 0 9 9 6 8 8 6 0 0 0 *